BARR[Y]

YOU A[RE]

REAL COURAGE...

BILL WOODARD

Barry, what you & Karen are
doing for the youth of our
community is _so_ great it
goes beyond words I have.
Thank you. George Halkias

Barry, your journey has been
extraordinary and inspiring to
us all. Thanks for sharing
your story.
Randy Thompson

YOU'RE DIGNIFIED FIGHT AGAINST
THIS MONSTER WE CALL PARKINSONS
HAS BEEN INSPIRING TO ME. YOU
HAVE HELPED ME TO UNDERSTAND IT
BETTER THEN ANY TEXT BOOK - THANK YOU
[signature] LPN

Dad,
Thank you for
sharing your struggles
with Parkinson's
disease! This will
help me to fight
this ugly beast just
in case I get it
        Love always,
            Jennifer

Many will be blessed that you
have shared your story about your
journey with this disease; that you
have had so much courage and will
is to be admired!
        ~ Michelle

Barry, I am so glad
I have got to know
you and Karen. I love
how you keep going
And it makes me do
the same - BethAnn Smith

Barry, Here's looking to + trusting (by faith) that in Heaven there is no pain! Glory

Thank you for sharing your story with me! You have been an inspiration to me and I am honored to get to work with you! God Bless You! *Jennifer Pey*

Barry - an honor to get to know too and read Description of something special to share

IT NEVER STOPS TAKING

Parkinsons—The Undefeated

Thank you Barry for the opportunity to know such a hero + patriot. You are truely the undefeated. *Tina Venn*

BARRY W. LOWE

Barry, very happy that you accomplished this book. It is quite remarkable. All the best, *Jeff Martindale, Ph.D.*

Mr. Lowe It is a pleasure working for you & thank you for the book, can't wait to Read it.

iUniverse, Inc.
Bloomington

It Never Stops Taking
Parkinsons—The Undefeated

iUniverse books may be ordered through booksellers or by contacting:

iUniverse
1663 Liberty Drive
Bloomington, IN 47403
www.iuniverse.com
1-800-Authors (1-800-288-4677)

ISBN: 978-1-4759-2686-6 (sc)
ISBN: 978-1-4759-2692-7 (ebk)

Printed in the United States of America

iUniverse rev. date: 06/07/2012

To my beloved wife, Karen, who typed and retyped the manuscript and supports me in the bad times.

To my father, Wilbur, and my sister, Sharon Joy, who suffered with Parkinson's.

To Bill Woodard, my best friend, who stood with me when others wouldn't.

To Pastor Rod MacIlvaine and Sheryl Kaufman, who reviewed the manuscript with a different perspective.

To my beloved cousin Virginia, whose father suffered through many years with Parkinson's.

To my friend Kimberly, who did the art work for the front and back covers.

Real courage is … when you know you're licked before you begin but you begin anyway and you see it through no matter what.

Harper Lee, *To Kill a Mockingbird*

Contents

FOREWORD

When Barry Lowe started publishing his journal as e-mails to a few friends, I was better acquainted with Parkinson's disease than I was with Barry. Through following the story of his experience as the disease progressed, I learned to know him better as a person, an engineer, and a scientist. His careful, almost dispassionate, observations of himself as patient and the care available to him are certainly as close to the "real world as laboratory" as the medical community will ever find.

Barry pulls no punches. Parkinson's is a devastating disease that slowly eats away a person's capabilities to a level where the core of dignity is redefined. There is no standing on pretenses when merely standing is an "iffy" proposition.

My father struggled with Parkinson's the last several years of his life. He endured not only loss of control of his limbs, but also, possibly more frustrating, loss of feedback as to whether those limbs were, or even had, done what he believed his mind had directed.

Loss of control is probably more aggravating to an engineer than to most personalities. Thus, I admired Barry for seizing control of his story even as he lost control of the plot.

He determined to capture the story in detail, and now he is ready to share it with a wider audience. The final chapters are not yet unfolded, and I believe Barry knows that his ability to record them will be increasingly limited. Whether you are reading this as a patient, a caregiver, or a friend, this journal will help you understand—and perhaps conquer—this disease by controlling it in your own way.

Sheryl Kaufman
Chief Economist
Phillips Petroleum Company, Retired

PREFACE

It Never Stops Taking was never intended to become a book. Writing allowed me to keep my sanity during a very difficult time in my life. Writing was an outlet for my innermost emotions.

In 2002, I lost my mother, my father, and my mother-in-law in a 13-week period. All of them were elderly. Mom suffered a heart attack, went into a coma and her 3 children made the decision to remove her from life support. My mother-in-law died next from total renal failure. My father had surgery to remove an aortic aneurysm. He was in intensive care for eight weeks before his children decided to have the life support removed. He died 13 weeks after his wife.

During this string of losses, I was in my fourth year of Parkinson's. I had started to use the Internet and had become more knowledgeable about this disease. Two facts were apparent. First, Parkinson's never lost. Second, the average life span after one is diagnosed is 11 years.

I was fulfilling my traditional role as the alpha male when nine months later, Kris (my wife of 31 years) and I and two friends were in an automobile accident. Kris was killed immediately. Our two friends suffered broken ribs and other injuries. I didn't have a scratch. After this loss, I was a total wreck.

As my Parkinson's gained strength and my memory deteriorated, I used my diary to talk to Kris, and I also used it to keep track of all of my medications. I had already learned that there was no standard treatment for Parkinson's, and the best drug for slowing the progress of the disease was developed back in 1973. Put another way, in the preceding three decades, there had been no significant research results on curing Parkinson's disease.

In less than the course of a year, I had lost three close relatives and then my wife, my best friend. I had just about had it when the Lord gave me a helper. I never would have made it without her. Karen became my second wife.

I analyzed my personal data, including my responses to the various Parkinson's drugs. Doctors don't like to talk about Parkinson's—probably because there is no right answer. I have had seven neurologists who each had different opinions about treating Parkinson's. I have had major brain surgery to implant a medical device for a treatment called DBS, or deep brain stimulation. It slowed down the progression, but the disease continues to gain. Two doctors have told me they could not help me. I asked several nurses, "Where are the patients who have had Parkinson's for 11 years or more?" They told me that the patients were all in nursing homes.

There are some drug treatments that alleviate some symptoms of Parkinson's, but these have side effects as well.

There is agreement that using Sinemet—the primary drug for Parkinson's—can increase your risk of falling. In the last two years, I have had four broken ribs, two dislocated thumbs, two torn rotator cuffs, and one dislocated shoulder. That really hurt. In all, I've also had 35 stitches and staples, a brain hemorrhage that required emergency surgery, and assorted contusions of varying severity.

The intent of providing this record of several years in my journey is to make you aware of the challenges that a person with Parkinson's must live with. At this journey's end you will understand the feeling of going to bed each night knowing that when you wake up the next morning you will be as stiff as a board, you will need assistance to get out of bed, you will need help to put on your shoes and socks, you will need help to take a shower.

Such is the life of a Parkinsonian.

INTRODUCTION

Barry Lowe is one of the most remarkable men I've ever met.

I got to know Barry several years ago when he and his new fiancée came to me for premarital counseling.

A retired oil company executive and an engineering specialist, Barry had endured the worst kind of tragedy. His wife of 31 years was killed in a car wreck. The offending driver was a sixteen-year-old who'd just received her license.

Barry was devastated, no doubt, but Barry set up a meeting between himself and the driver, with intent to offer forgiveness, provided the driver got "to know" his deceased wife.

At the meeting, Barry showed old pictures. He regaled her with stories about Kris and the richness of their family. They both shed tears. And in the aftermath of the meeting, Barry offered his forgiveness, and he went on with his life, eventually marrying again and starting a new life with fresh purpose.

I kept discovering surprising things about Barry.

He was an active member of the local school board and

quite passionate about education. Not only was he creative in leading the board, but he was also willing to personally invest in the education of students in his community. Because Barry grew up in poverty, he committed to help the children of the working poor get a good education. Along with his new wife, Karen, they founded the Lowe Family Young Scholars Foundation, a unique mentoring program for students of financially challenged families, designed especially for needy students from 8th through 11th grade.

Barry and Karen put up a huge portion of their net worth, and then obtained matching funds from other organizations, so that qualified kids who could never afford college on their own had a chance. They also recruited mentors, community partners and educational specialists to assist them in their cause. Five years later, there is a growing collection of Lowe Family Scholars who are excelling in college, landing strong jobs, and pursuing degrees in graduate education.

Barry was inspired by the example of his father, and now Barry leaves a lasting legacy to children of the working poor in Bartlesville, Oklahoma, whose fathers could never provide them with a college degree.

And I kept discovering more surprising things about Barry.

Barry is a fighter. He's like the boxer who stays in the ring no matter how many times he's been knocked down, just so he can outlast his opponent. When he was diagnosed with Parkinson's disease, he didn't give in or give up. Rather, he did what Barry typically does; he fought to live the best life he could under extremely challenging circumstances.

In the early phase of his illness, he plunged into researching the disease. Ransacking medical journals, medical textbooks and Internet sites, Barry gained a broad knowledge of his illness, and therefore was able to challenge conventional thinking. His doctors were surprised at his growing knowledge and his willingness to explore fresh treatment options. Whereas others were giving up, Barry was back on his feet ready to try something new.

When there were setbacks, he never let the dark cloud of Parkinson's knock him into a corner of despair. On the contrary, his sparkling sense of humor endeared him his to caregivers and friends alike. As a result, Barry Lowe, 13 years into his illness, is still on his feet, sometimes even able to muster a smile on his face, even in the advanced stages of his illness. Many of his contemporaries with fewer years in the disease are languishing in nursing homes.

Barry's tenacity in fighting Parkinson's makes him an encouraging guide for those who've just been diagnosed with the disease. Barry's heroism in fighting Parkinson's makes him a trustworthy model that anyone struggling with Parkinson's will appreciate. If you are seeking an honest manual for how to think and function with this disease, I believe this is the ideal place to begin.

Most of you who read this book won't have the privilege of knowing Barry as I know him: a man with a big heart for students in need, a man willing to forgive the teen who took the life of his first wife, a man who is at home leading a school board and serving at the highest levels of a Fortune 500 company, and a man still passionate about "his" scholars.

But what you will get to know about Barry in this book is his soldier spirit. He is an inspiration for those willing to take this disease by the horns and fight back.

Barry's courage has inspired me personally (someone

without the disease) to be stretched a bit more, and trust my Creator with greater tenacity, knowing that He has the power to sustain me through any trial I might face.

Rod MacIlvaine, D.Min.
Fellow, Veritas Center for Faith, Freedom and Justice,
  Oklahoma Wesleyan University
Senior Pastor, Grace Community Church, Bartlesville,
  Oklahoma

PART I

Background to the Diary

I came into this world on April 9, 1945, born to a couple who experienced hard times in their lives and who would raise me in one of the poorest communities in the United States. I was fortunate enough, however, to inherit my father's quiet intelligence. Also, both of my parents' hard-work ethics were innately enmeshed in my genes. This caused me to push myself, a youngster growing up in the small coal-mining community of Pottsville, Pennsylvania, to be the best that I could be.

In my preteen and teenage years, I often came home from school, ate my dinner in solitude as my parents were both at work, washed the family dishes, studied until 9:30 or 10:00 p.m. each evening, and went to bed. It was a lonely existence, but I knew nothing else. I was being prepared for my life.

As a high school sophomore, I desperately wanted to succeed in academics so I could win the only scholarship given to a student body selection of around 300 students. I ended up quitting a promising football career to focus on my studies. Due to my intense drive and motivation, I was in the hospital for a short bout with an ulcer. Yes, the pressure was on, but I was learning how to handle it. I was being prepared for my life.

After receiving the one community scholarship, I attended Lafayette college and majored in chemical engineering. I had the rug pulled out from under me as the college started pulling funds from my scholarship. I joined the ROTC—for the money—and worked as the treasurer for my fraternity so I could eat. In addition to working at least 20 hours a week, I studied 20 hours a week and was going to class another 30-40 hours a week.

It was rough, but I completed my stint at Lafayette through

sheer grit and determination. I hated my time there because of the stress that controlled my life and because they removed my promised scholarship funds. I remember one particular time when I sat in class and I was so exhausted, so totally depleted, that my mind went blank. I was taking a test and all I could do was write my name on the paper and turn it in blank. Failure, however, was not an option, and this challenge did not consume me. I was being prepared for my life. I graduated.

After college, I worked for six months at Proctor & Gamble and then went into the Army to complete my two year commitment from ROTC. The first 16 months I was in El Paso where I met my future wife Kris. I became a combat infantry adviser and was sent to Vietnam. I led others. Waving a flag of surrender was not an option. I do not give up.

During this time in Vietnam, I was exposed to Agent Orange, an herbicide-defoliant that the US military sprayed there. Agent Orange was declared presumptive to Parkinson's Disease in 2010.

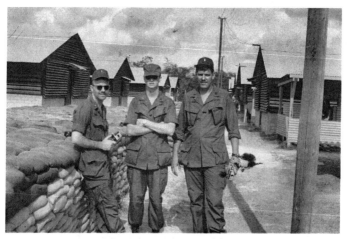

Barry's Vietnam Buddies

I came back alive. I am amazed that I survived this chapter of my life. God must have had a plan for my life. I did survive, but my worst enemy was not the one that I could see and return fire; it was one that perhaps was there, lying dormant, when the exposure to Agent Orange ignited it and brought it to life. I brought my worst enemy home with me. I would battle it for many years. There would be no cease fire. It would never surrender. But I don't surrender easily either.

Returning to civilian living, I married Kris, the love of my life, and we had two beautiful daughters. I had a promising career as a project manager for a major oil company. I knew how to find solutions to tough problems. I was a fixer. I did not accept defeat easily.

Near the end of my successful career of 31 years, in 1998, I noticed a foot dragging; the heel was worn out on one shoe. I walked with a limp. My arm wasn't swinging fully. All of this was on the same side of my body. I had a suspicion.

There were no neurologists in town, but my primary care physician concluded that my limp was due to lower back surgery and my arm problem was due to upper back surgery. There was moderate arthritis and some scar tissue. I had back pain almost constantly.

At about this time, my sister learned she had Parkinson's Disease. She didn't have tremors but had other symptoms. I started researching and decided that I could also have Parkinson's.

In the year 2001, a neurologist moved into town. He determined that I had Parkinson's by watching me walk 20 feet. He gave me pills for Parkinson's Disease, and my back pain went away within 48 hours.

My dad had Parkinson's. I had an uncle who had it and

my sister had already been diagnosed with it earlier. As I came to grips with having Parkinson's, I thought this must have been why I had been tested and hardened by life's challenges. I would now use what I had learned in my earlier life lessons to fight PD. God, however, has other plans. The lessons were not over.

Not long after this, I lost my mother, my mother-in-law, my father, and then my partner—my wife, Kris—in a short time frame. I felt like the biblical Job. Many close to me whom I dearly loved were removed from my life. My mind screamed out, "God, are the lessons over with *now?*" I'm vulnerable, I'm tough, but I was feeling a bit defeated. This was another life lesson. God is in control. He was not through with me yet and even though I had PD, He was not prepared to let me surrender. He had a plan for my life, and I still had to fight.

He soon allowed me to meet my second wife, Karen, who would fight this battle with me.

Maybe it took all of these life events to put me in a place where I could accept that God is in control and that He had a purpose for my life that was so much bigger than my disease or me. He made it quite plain to me that I was to give up a huge amount of my personal wealth to aid students whose families needed assistance with college expenses. Hence, the Lowe Family Young Scholars Program was born. To date, we have many students being academically mentored in preparation of receiving college scholarships.

As to my Parkinson's Disease, when my first neurologist stopped practicing in town, we found a Dr. Hastings in Tulsa, about 50 miles away. He was super. In our first meeting he talked with my wife, Karen, and me for four hours. He changed my medication. I was probably Stage 2 and was still very active. I became involved in a Parkinson's support group and was prescribed a new drug called Azilect. The label said you could die from a heart attack while taking this drug. The doctor said I was the only one of his patients willing to take the risk. Also, he introduced me to a doctor in Houston who was a world-renowned expert in Parkinson's. The first thing that doctor did was change my medications.

This rang an alarm bell—three different doctors and three different medications. The doctor also told me that the best Parkinson's drug had been developed in 1973 and that nothing better had been found since. There was no cure.

Eventually I decided I had to get more involved with my own treatment. I started keeping records of my medications and my reaction to them. I started this in 2006 and I am continuing to keep records today. It has been very helpful, especially when I get a new neurologist. From 2001 to 2006 they had used a stew of pills, trying to find a mix that would give a longer average cycle time. (Cycle time is the period between flare-ups of symptoms or between dosings of medication.) There was lots of trial and error. In my diary you will see that a person with Parkinson's can have an active lifestyle in Stages 1 and 2 but not in Stages 4 and 5. I am in Stage 5 and my activities are severely limited. My first doctor told me I would have 20 years before I was impaired. He was wrong.

A major challenge is the different methods of treatment. After one has tried all the drugs, the only option is surgery to install a device that sends electrical impulses to the brain. It is called Deep Brain Stimulation—DBS. The operation takes four and a half hours. Using the DBS system may give the person a longer cycle time. If the surgery doesn't work, the person suffers more. I had mixed success with DBS.

After DBS, a person with Parkinson's is back to trying different drugs to find the combination that will give the best cycle time. My cycle time is now two and a half hours. I take the following pills: Sinemet, Azilect, Neupro, Lotrel, and Provigil. To be effective, the primary medications for Parkinson's must be taken several times per day, at precise intervals—sometimes every two or three hours. In addition, as the years pass, the effectiveness of some of the drugs diminishes in a particular user. It can be a continuing pursuit to identify drugs and dosages that work well together and that support the effectiveness of the primary drug used for Parkinson's, called levodopa.

In my case, the Parkinson's has progressed and has been currently diagnosed as "Stage 5" or "advanced Parkinson's Disease." Sometimes I can walk. Sometimes I freeze in place and cannot move. Some days I am confined to a wheel chair all day long. At night, I become stiff as a log and have to have a night attendant who will move me from side to side to loosen me up. He gets me up to take pills at four o'clock every morning. Also, I have to wear a catheter at night due to severe incontinence.

My diary tells my journey during recent years. It shares my frustrations and battles. Parkinson's is a worthy adversary, and frankly, it will win in the end. However, I will fight the good battle.

Through my diary entries, you will get a glimpse of my life over the past five years or so. I'm engaged in life; I didn't check out with my diagnosis. I continued to serve on the school board, attend events, remain active.

This is my encouragement to others: Don't give in to the disease. Fight it with every ounce of strength. I've been likened to a boxer in a boxing ring with an opponent who is much stronger and bigger and who I know will eventually knock me out and win the battle, yet I stay in the ring. I take my punches and knock him backward a few times, however, I know, deep in my heart, this opponent will eventually win. Yet I tell myself, "I don't care; I must fight the battle as though I could have a chance." That is what my life lessons have taught me … to never give up … even if my opponent is Parkinson's Disease.

PART II

Diary of a Parkinsonian

This part of the book contains selections from the diary I kept, starting with entries from 2006. Also included are portions of correspondence to or from friends and relatives and my medical team. I distributed parts of my diary via e-mail postings. The diary excerpts shown here have been proofread and styled for publication and to make their meaning clear. The diary may contain some factual inaccuracies or inconsistencies, as I was not always at my literary best when writing it. Where necessary, I included explanatory notations in this version.

April 7, 2006—Medications
[These were my medications when I first started keeping a written record.]

- Stalevo

- Requip

- Provigil

- Clonazepam

- Seroquel for hallucinations; try Clonazepam in place of Seroquel.

- Still on Lotrel, Pyrodostigimine, hydrochlorothiazide, Celebrex

- Results—Reduced Provigil did not work.

- Stopped Selegeline, amantadine, Artane.

June 20, 2006—Medications
- Stopped amantadine.

- Stopped Selegeline HCL.

- Still on Stalevo, Provigil, Celebrex, Pyrodostigimine, Artane
- Finish Artane and go to Requip.

August 2006—Medications

- Lotrel
- Stalevo
- Provigil
- Hydrochlorothiazide
- Requip
- Clonazepam
- Artane
- Celebrex
- Seroquel
- Pyrodostigimine

March 14, 2007—Medications

- Adjust Artane to 5x day.
- Adjust Stalevo.
- Eliminate Pyrodostigimine.

March 21, 2007—Medications

- Remove Requip.

April 5, 2007—Medications

- Remove Artane and every other Stalevo.

April 11, 2007—Medications

- Add Artane back, take Stalevo dosage every time.

June 8, 2007—Medications

- Keep Artane, keep Azilect, replace Stalevo with Sinemet.

September 16, 2007—Activities Report

I arrived at the lake house on Wednesday. On Friday, I awoke at 7:30 and started to work at 8:00 a.m. My goal was to leave at noon; I didn't make it. My activities included:

- Repair the waterline from the lake. Temperature was 70 degrees. A big drop from 95. Plastic shrinks and the clamps are not tight. Need water to burn pit safely.

- Complete mowing the yard.

- Put more wire on the deck railing to prevent Braden from falling through.

- Write work order for polyethylene pipe to be installed in the guest cabin. Approximately 30–40 dead hornets were found inside. Vacuumed them up. Put water in the water traps.

- Write work scope for putting sun shield on the main deck.

- Wash dirty linens and clothes.

- No time to ride boat; put on canvas boat cover. Big log was not on the dock cable today.

- Loaded Tahoe. Completed by 1:30 p.m. Battery was dead. Kmart suggested that if rear door is left open, it will kill the battery. I think Kmart was right. Left Kmart at 2:30.

- On the way home, I dropped off contract documents; arrived home at 5:00 p.m.

- Left at 6:00 p.m. for Baptist Church picnic.

- Went to high school homecoming at 7:30 p.m. Lost to Stillwater.

- Arrived at two-steppers at 9:00 p.m. Left at 11:00 p.m.

- Fell asleep quickly (16-hour day—no rest for the wicked).

September 20, 2007—Medications

Following are my current medications:

- Azilect

- Provigil

- Sinemet

- Hydrochlorothiazide

- Celebrex

- Seroquel

- Clonazepam

- Stopped Lotrel.

September 28, 2007—
Activities Report/Medical Condition

The last 48 hours have seen high highs and new lows. The highs first: Karen and I were awarded "Citizen of the Year" by the local Civitan Club. It was a surprise and very nice. Today we gave Jane Phillips School the glass eagle paper weight awards for achieving an API of 1451. Karen did all the work. It is a beautiful glass eagle with an inscription.

The lows now: Last night I had my first freeze. After the Civitan dinner, I made it to the truck, but had to hold on.

October 3, 2007—
Activities Report/Drug Explanation

My meds were working pretty well until 4:40 p.m. When we went to the driving range, I was terrible. Then, went to a new Mexican restaurant for margaritas and nachos. It was a great day until the meds wore off. I could barely walk. Took some more and was better by 8:00 p.m. I told Karen that sometimes I wonder why I have had to bear so much pain and heartache the past five years. I told her that without her I would not have made it. It is true.

I have been thinking of how to explain the cycles of PD by using a sine wave. Basically, a typical sine wave would be this:

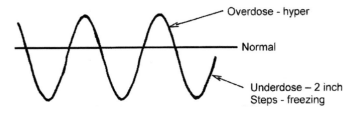

Typical Medication Cycle

When I take Sinemet 25/100 [a pill with 25 mg of the drug carbidopa and 100 mg of levodopa], the cycle is two hours to two hours 30 minutes long. It takes one half hour to ramp up. That is good for two hours and then it drops off like an electric switch. Not good.

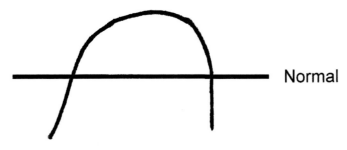

Barry's Normal Cycle

When I take a Sinemet 25/250, it ramps up for an hour, and depending on when it follows a 25/100, I can quickly go into a real overdose situation or severe under dose.

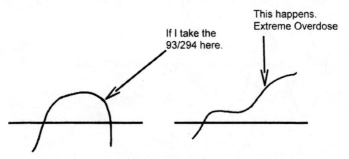

Extreme Overdose

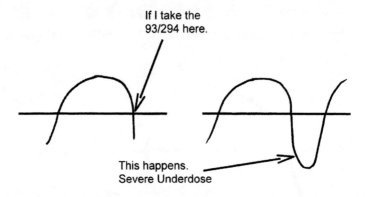

Severe Under Dose

My problem is exaggerated because my body reacts very quickly to drugs. I had a "happy pill" before back surgery one time and it put me out—it took four orderlies to put me on the gurney.

October 7, 2007—Activities/Medications

We had planned to go to the zoo but didn't make it. We spent three hours with Bud, Marlene, Dean, and Ryan. They are a neat family. We visited with my son-in-law, Cliff. He looked much better with a full night's rest (he works night shifts as a policeman).

Braden is almost walking. He likes everyone, sleeps at night, says "Dada" all the time. We are working on him to say "Momma." He did it once. He eats like a horse. We had spaghetti and applesauce at my mother-in-law's home.

I continue trying to get the right amount of Sinemet. I have stopped taking three drugs: Artane, Clonazepam, and Selegeline. Sometimes the meds wear off very quickly. Just took meds at 6:00 p.m.—will wear off during the symphony. It could be interesting.

October 18, 2007—
Activities/Medical Condition

We went to the family cottage in Pennsylvania. Looked good; Tommy is doing a good job improving the cottage. Karen and I walked around the lake. We talked about Mom and Dad. Karen found another penny.

Next, we visited Aunt Rosetta and George (her son-in-law). She will be 82 shortly. She had skin cancer on her legs. It was nice to visit her.

Next we traveled to see Sharon [my sister]. We worked out deed information. She is slipping; she had a lump on her neck. Sharon went to the doctor in the morning, and it was gone! They will do a CT scan. We watched my nephew's soccer game. Tommy went with us—that was good. We enjoyed submarine sandwiches at Sharon and Ned's house. Dixie is their new dog. Emma (their previous dog) had to be put asleep. Dixie eats ice and is very friendly.

During this trip, I had another PD experience. Just before

the trip, we changed my medications to try to extend the good part of the cycle. I was taking four Stalevo and went to five.

November 21, 2007—
Symptoms, Medications, and Side Effects

- Two Sinemet 25/100's last 2 hours 15 minutes.

- One-half of a Sinemet 25/250 lasts 1 hour 45 minutes.

- I cannot take one Sinemet 25/250 in a.m. or during the day—goes late into overdose symptoms.

- I can adjust two Sinemet25/100's or one-half Sinemet 25/250 to match meeting schedule.

- If I go too long one Sinemet 25/100 works; one Sinemet 25/250 puts me in an overdose in an hour—cold sweats.

- Meals reduce time by 50 percent.

- Works pretty good. I must hit times. Sitting down—don't realize I miss times until standing up.

- Constipation continues to be a problem.

- Urinate 6x during sleep time.

- Blood pressure up to 145/90. Was 120/70.

- Balance is a problem at times.

- If eat fruits and vegetables—same as cheese and meat.

- I expect the 24-hour patch will help.

- How do we know Azilect is working? It will extend the effective time of Sinemet.

- Why only two Provigil? Provigil is a controlled substance—may become addictive.

- Does chocolate cause problems?
- Should I go back to Lotrel? Yes, November 22.

November 29, 2007— Medications/Medical Team

- Will start on 24-hour patch of Neupro. There are some potential side effects.
- Dr. Hastings will refer me to Dr. Jankovich who is regarded as a world-class expert in research for PD.

December 4, 2007—Sleepiness Issues

I have decided not to use the 24-hour patch. A major side effect is falling asleep with no warning. Twice before when I changed medication, I had some episodes. With Requip I fell asleep four times [I nodded off momentarily while driving] in the 50 miles between Tulsa and Bartlesville. Also, when driving home from the lake, I stopped to sleep in a convenience store parking lot. I was awakened by the sheriff and several deputies. They said I had been asleep for two hours. I also fell asleep in an Oklahoma School Board Association meeting in Oklahoma City. Plus, the 24-hour patch raises blood pressure. Three to four months after I discontinued Lotrel, my blood pressure went up to 145/92. After going back to Lotrel I went back to my normal 120/75.

December 28, 2007— Medications/Medical Issues

My current medications:
- Sinemet—18 pills; 1 per waking hour

- Provigil—2
- Azilect—1
- Celebrex—1
- Lotrel—1
- Fibercon—4
- Seroquel—1
- Cutting back on Provigil. Eventually to go to zero if possible.
- Move Celebrex from evening to dinner time—should take with food.
- Are 18 Sinemet 25/100's per day bad?

Had another episode today. Get totally weak and dizzy. High blood pressure—150/95.

It's getting late, I cannot write very well. My dream Mustang is happy. [I purchased a special 2008 Mustang with 465 hp and a Roush supercharger on all forward gears.] I was raised in a poor neighborhood, worked my way through college, worked 60 hours a week at my job, and donated approximately $1,000,000. to others. This was the first time I bought something special for myself. Everyone said I deserved to get it.

April 11, 2008—Activities/Medications

Last weekend we spent two days and one night at the lake. Everything went well. Jennafer has great patience with the two boys and I am surprised and pleased. I could not do it. Melissa is happy to be pregnant. She is having a daughter whom they will name Kristy after her mother. Melissa's husband, Johnny, expects to have a transfer to Tulsa by the first of May. They are looking for a house with 2.5 acres. Cliff (Jennafer's husband) is still with the Tulsa Police Department and feels good about it. He is also working part time as a security guard. I have two good daughters and two good son-in-laws but I rarely see them.

I have had a running battle with Social Security. They said PD was not a disability. I appealed with gusto, and now I will receive $2,200 per month.

- Medication has changed recently. Neupro (24-hour patch) was pulled from the market due to manufacturing problems.

- Dr. Ferrara (Dr. Jankovich's office)—I tried to stop 6 mg Neupro and replace it with 5 mg Requip. This did not work well. I felt really terrible after taking the Requip twice per day.

- We decided to cut Neupro to 3 mg per day and increase Sinemet if necessary.

- I have increased Sinemet from two Sinemet 25/100's to one Sinemet 25/250 twice per day.

- The increased dosage has not lengthened the cycle. Still at two hours. If I go two hours to two hours and 15 minutes, I have underdose symptoms for 30–45 minutes. I must take pills every two hours.

- I have not had high blood pressure excursions (165/110) in some time. My normal blood pressure is still 125/75. In fact I had 125/75 before the nasal surgery and the other day it was 96/68.

- I must start thinking seriously about deep brain stimulation. What is the proper time to try this?

- Sharon, my sister, is doing so much better after they took her off the antidepressant drug. Her speech is almost perfect.

April 25, 2008–Activities/Nasal Surgery

A lot has happened. I have begun to write my diary. I was at the lake by myself for a few days. Two weeks ago I had a new heat pump installed in the main lake house. I don't plan to start any more major projects at the lake. One day I lay in the hammock for 20 minutes and then took the boat out for a run. Maybe I'm learning to relax and enjoy.

Guess I should include this: I was recognized as Progressive Citizen of the Year. It felt good to be recognized by the citizens of Bartlesville, but I get embarrassed when respected adults tell me they are honored to meet me. It was an honor to be selected but I had a lot of others who helped me.

More people seem to be aware of the challenge to be an effective president of the school board with advanced Parkinson's. Getting seven very independent individuals to work together, with the restrictions of the Open Meeting Act, was difficult. I stepped down as president after four years due to the increased demands of PD and my desire to spend more time with Karen. It was gratifying to be able to lead real change in the district that resulted in significantly improved test scores and hopefully better education.

April 2 was our wedding anniversary. Karen wanted to get away, and she planned everything. We went to Kansas City and stayed at a downtown Hilton. I saw my first 3-D movie, *Monsters of the Deep*. It was very realistic. We searched and searched for a rodeo museum that we had read about. Nobody was there. We got in for free. Karen and I were being kids again.

I took the Mustang to Hallet (an Oklahoma race track) for a day of racing. It was great—three sessions of running 15 minutes at a time. I was terrible but am improving. My best lap time was 2 minutes 2 seconds. A teenager who rented a racer for the first time ran 1 minute 30 seconds. I go into the turns too fast—too much horsepower—then I had to brake like crazy.

I had nasal surgery on April 11. Dr. Mark Robertson worked on my nose for two hours. I was plenty sore the first three days and still am not fully healed. I honestly thought I might die during the nasal surgery and God had given me time to get my affairs in order. My affairs are okay and He let me stay on.

April 28, 2008—Symptoms/Medications

I woke up later than normal and took my first pills at 9:00 a.m. I had PD symptoms ten minutes later. I took a second Sinemet 25/100 at 11:00 a.m. and had overdose symptoms through the Rotary lunch, so I delayed the next dose until 2:20 p.m., just before a doctor's appointment. Ten minutes later I had stutter steps for an hour. I took a Sinemet 25/250 at 3:00 p.m. Went home, still had symptoms. Went to bed, had dinner and still could not walk. Sat down in the den and fell asleep. I woke up stiff as a board. I took a Sinemet 25/100 at 7:30 p.m., which didn't help. I took a Sinemet 25/250 at eight. Finally, about 9:00 p.m. I could walk. It was a crappy day. I have never been able to take just one Sinemet 25/100—don't know why. Sinemet 25/100 pills on their own give me all kinds of problems.

May 1, 2008—Medications Dosage

Today I really tried to watch my two-hour limit. It was better, but not good enough. In fact, I took a second dosage ten minutes early, but it did not help. Also, I worked in the yard. Physical labor uses up pills quicker. I took one Sinemet one hour after the last dosage and another Sinemet two hours after. This pill schedule seems to work, but I still get baby steps 15 minutes after I take pills. I don't understand. I'm still on Neupro. Need to go off totally soon. Maybe the Neupro shortened the start-up time.

May 6, 2008—Medications Dosage

Once again, shortly after I took my second dose at 10:00 a.m., I went gaga. No walk, no talk. Went to bed. Symptoms lasted for two hours even though I had put on a 24-hour patch. Took another Sinemet at ten-thirty. Today I was going off the patch, but it didn't work. The patch eliminated the depth of the lows. It appears the lows are back without the patch. I will call. The majority of the time—15 minutes after I take Sinemet—I have PD symptoms for 30–45 minutes.

May 15, 2008—
Activities/Medical Consultation

Karen and I had massages, went to lunch, and toured the Dewey hotel, which was built in the 1890s.

I talked with Dr. Joseph Ferrara on Wednesday. We decided to stop Neupro patch. I mentioned how quickly the on/off switch is working. Also, the meds do not seem to be working at times.

On Monday I had 11 hours of down time: nine hours with two-step and two hours of bob and weave. I was a little better yesterday until late night. From 9:00 p.m. to 3:00 a.m. I really felt terrible.

I looked at a website where Melissa bought my vibrating pager. It is a very good site. I ordered three other types of alarms. I need to be on schedule for taking pills.

Dr. Ferrara and I decided as follows:

- Stop using Neupro.

- Increase Sinemet.

- Make appointment with Dr. Jankovich to begin investigation into surgery for Deep Brain Stimulation.

- Only one drug option remains. That is to add Mirapex. We will discuss that at our next appointment.

- I am to bring down the brain scans.

- Make appointment ASAP.

May 23, 2008—Activities/Medications

Karen went to Oklahoma City for a bachelorette party for Megan. She drove to Bartlesville on Saturday afternoon. We left for the lake at 1:30 p.m. At the lake we met Melissa and Zoe. Melissa is quite pregnant. Karen and I left at 1:30 to host Marlene's 75th birthday. Marlene, Bud, Dean, Dana, Frank, Brad, Ryan, Karen attended. It was a very good holiday.

My current cycle time is 1 hour 45 minutes with 225 mg of Sinemet.

May 23, 2008—Caregiver Discussion

Karen gave up Mary Martha Outreach volunteer work, and I gave up country dancing and going to college football and basketball games. Anyway, while she had described her dream of helping lots of people significantly, this leaves less time for me. Also, as my PD gets worse, I will be responsible for her not achieving her dream. I will not do that. When she asked me what my dream was, I said I don't have one. She said, "What about the school board and the Lowe Family Young Scholars Program?"

May 25, 2008—Medications Schedule

Target Pill Taking Time	Actual Pill Taking Time
7:30	7:40
9:15	9:00
11:00	11:10
12:45	1:30
2:30	3:00
4:15	4:15
6:00	6:00
7:45	7:45

With Karen and Melissa's help, plus two vibrating watches, I was pretty much on time. One of the best days I have had in a while. I even worked outside some.

June 2, 2008—Correspondence
To: Pastor Rod

Rod, I thought your sermon today was excellent. May I have a copy? Also, I would like to share a few thoughts with you that do scare me.

First, there are times in church when I feel like there is a presence inside me, a presence that makes me even more compassionate than normal. I have always cried at funerals, at movies where pure emotions such as love, courage, fear, etc., are presented. I cried at *Old Yeller*, and *A Clockwork Orange* made me mad as hell, but this feeling is much bigger. It is hard to explain.

In the last three years, I have received praise and recognition and awards far beyond what I deserve. So many people come to me and tell me what an honor it is to meet me, etc. I have told Karen that I don't deserve such. Karen and I have told many gatherings that we believe God has put us together to help children. When we run into an obstacle, an answer is just around the corner. A lady told us the other day that she was waiting for God to give her a challenge to help others and our program was His answer. I have been told many times how I have inspired others. I am not that good. It scares me that intelligent people say these things and appear to mean them.

For quite some time, I have believed that God has guided my life in a fashion to prepare me for what I am currently doing. I have had 22 close calls with death. I was in the infantry, but not wounded. I believe He took my mother, father, and mother-in-law in 13 weeks to clear the decks, so to speak. The pain was almost unbearable. It caused me to find it inconceivable how any man could bear the pain of mankind's sins that Jesus did on the cross, but Jesus was not a man, He is God.

But the loss of these three did not change my life. Kris, my wonderful wife and partner and was part of my soul, who would do anything for anyone, had a different direction for me. She wanted to travel after retirement, but God did not want my life to take this path, so He took Kris away. I am convinced she is in heaven. The pain of her leaving almost killed me. I believe God knew I was too weak to carry any burden, so He sent Karen to me.

I fell in love so quickly, but I did not feel I was disrespectful of my love for Kris. All of my friends understood and were very supportive, and some are very picky. And then God sent us to deliver Thanksgiving baskets, which planted the seed for the Lowe Family Young Scholars Program. This was a pivotal point in my life.

I feel like I am now an instrument to do God's will. Is this vanity? Just saying these words scares me.

People say I am humble; I know that is not true, but I also know I am not as good as many say.

Response From: Pastor Rod

Barry, your words were such an encouragement to me that I had to read them several times and think about them before answering you.

Your perspective on your suffering and pain is so healthy and so correct.

I am thankful to see someone processing his "story" the way you are doing it. I can't imagine the pain you went through. Cindy's mother is dying of cancer right now. Cindy is traveling to see her this coming week. I see the pain she is in, and I can't imagine the pain you went through. And yet, by God's grace, he's led you in a direction that brings good out of the pain. Moreover, this direction honors the memory of your wider family, including your parents and Kris.

What a blessing to be able to take hurt and pain and bring meaning and purpose out of it.

I also am thankful for the example of Karen and how she works with you in your efforts to serve children in our community. I can see that the two of you have a sense of purpose that must seem larger than just the two of you.

Your work (along with Karen, of course) has brought people together to serve those in need. Your work has brought families together with goals and plans and a sense of purpose. Your work has encouraged the community to think creatively about how to make a difference.

I can truly see that both of you are instruments of God's work. I am thankful that you feel you don't deserve it. In so many ways we don't deserve the blessings we have. But you have been faithful to seize opportunities to serve and forge ahead in faith.

Barry you are a huge encouragement to me ... you and Karen both. Thank you for all you do to serve Christ.

June 13, 2008—Medications Effectiveness

- I've been taking Mirapex the last two weeks.
- I've been taking Sinemet CR for three weeks.
- I started amantadine on June 14.
- They seem to be having a positive effect. At night, I only wake up two to three times with four hours' sleep at a time. It used to be two hours' continuous sleep max. Also, I have been able to use a Sinemet 25/250.

June 22, 2008—Medications Effectiveness

I have reached a point where I can take three Mirapex per day and last week I started on amantadine twice per day.

I continue on Sinemet CR and Artane. I also continue to take Vesicare at bedtime. A summary of conclusions:

- The Vesicare has been effective at reducing urgency and incontinence.

- The Sinemet CR has given me four to six hours of uninterrupted sleep.

- I started the Mirapex first. It took two weeks to get amantadine. I also adjusted the Sinemet upward from one Sinemet 25/100 and one half a Sinemet 25/250 to one Sinemet 25/250 and one half a Sinemet 25/100.

- During the week of June 22–28, I had more bobbing and weaving than ever before. I decided to go to one Sinemet 25/250 for this week.

June 26, 2008—Daily Living with Parkinson's

I have a tendency to lose items I need for my daily existence such as my watch, my hearing aids, my reading glasses, my car keys, my pills, my hat. To stop losing all these items, I decided to put most of them in a fanny pack. (Not the hat!) What did I do the first day? I misplaced the fanny pack.

Mornings go well and then I forget. My watch only has six alarms: 7:30 a.m. to 5:30 p.m. I don't feel the buzzer when the buzzer is sitting on my clothes; it must have direct contact with my skin.

I will buy a second vibrating watch.

June 27, 2008—Activities/Functioning Ability

Today was a great day; probably the best day ever. Therefore no real stutter step or bobbing and weaving. It was a very busy day as well. I was up and out in the yard at 7:30 a.m. I went to Friday Financial Forum at ten o'clock. I drove to Tulsa for a talk sponsored by the PD Heartland of America. The guest speaker was Dr. Lawson. The talk was on DBS and gene therapy.

July 23, 2008—
Parkinson's Information/Activities/Caregiving

Today I was able to go greater than 2 hours 20 minutes between pills numerous times. I went to 2 hours 40 minutes and that was too much time between pills. I degraded to a stutter step for one hour. But what a good feeling—going from 1 hour 45 minutes to 2 hours 20 minutes—amazing how good that feels.

The day was normal with no major physical exertion.

I was disappointed with Friday's effort. I hit the first five medications on schedule, but around 1:30 p.m., I started two-stepping. It lasted until about 3:50 p.m. and then I forgot my interval and it was three hours before I realized I had missed a pill, but I was walking and talking like a normal person.

Karen and I are doing quite well together. As PD continues to make progress, she is becoming more of a caregiver. I don't like it, but I am very grateful. People know so little about PD. They think it is just shaking or being stiff. I am going to write up the other things that go on every day.

I experienced two severe reactions in the last month. Today I developed severe stomach pain, lots of gas that could not escape. I had cold sweats for an hour or more. For some period of time I could not move.

Karen helped me to bed. I was in bed for a short 15 minutes and she started putting on my socks. That was nice. Then she put on my underwear and then my shorts. I asked, "What am I getting dressed for?" She said, "We can still make a flight," and we did. I did not know I was well yet! She was determined not to miss her daughter's wedding.

A week ago I had the worst case of dizziness ever. Like six dimensions. Going left, going right, going up, going down, going fast, and going slow. It was awful. When you tell someone that you have PD, they understand you shake a lot or you get stiff and walk slow.

Now for the rest of the story.

I will list some of the side effects of PD and the drugs used to slow down PD. First, PD is a degenerative disease. It cannot be cured. PD kills most of its hosts by causing the host to fall. You lose something every day. You can fight it; you may be able to slow it down, but that is it. You go to bed at night knowing you will wake up in the morning feeling stiff as a board. You know you will have good and bad cycles. You know you will lose four to six hours per day when you go into a down cycle. You know if you sleep too late at night, it will take several hours to start the day. You may lose the entire day.

You schedule meetings, but you must warn people that you may not be able to come. You don't know when it will strike. You know that caring people will ask you how you feel. You don't say, "I have PD." I say, "I have a bad back," or something like that.

Yes, I have PD. I must live with it when I am awake and when I am asleep. What does PD do to me?

PD is a degenerative, incurable disease. It affects the entire body.

Symptom/Results of Parkinson's	My Personal Situation
All muscles will be constricted.	Yes, I'm very stiff.
Slow walking with head down.	Yes, every two-inch step hurts. That's why I don't smile.
Will lose balance.	I've fallen 5–6 times, broke 4 ribs, had 30 stitches and a subdural hematoma emergency brain surgery in the last 1½ years.
Will lose sense of smell.	I lost my sense of smell in 1967. It was approximately 30 years from when I lost smell to when I was diagnosed With PD.
Will experience significant back pain.	I've had significant pain for years. PD prevents muscles from relaxing. I always thought the pain was from back surgery. Two days after the first set of PD drugs, the back pain almost went all away. After 10-15 years, the drugs cannot lessen the pain.
Foot muscles are constricted.	I have developed three hammer toes because the muscles could not relax. I had to buy bigger and wider shoes.
Urinary incontinence	Yes, drip, drip drip.
Urinary urgency	Yes, when I have to go, I have to go right now! Sometimes I don't make it.
Poor sleep	Yes, up six times to urinate. Stiff body wakes me up after four hours.
Wake up with dry mouth.	Yes, 50 percent of the time, my tongue gets stuck on the roof of my mouth. Pills get stuck.
Nightmares	Yes, they are unbearable at times.

September 17, 2008—Medical Planning:
Deep Brain Stimulation (DBS)
To: Baylor College of Medicine

I have an appointment with Dr. Jankovich at 9:00 a.m. on Monday, November 3, 2008, and an appointment with Dr. Simpson at noon on the same day. Dr. Michele York informed me that I must take the On/Off Test first and this should be scheduled by your office at 9:00 a.m. that Monday.

Please verify this is correct or if I need to do something else. I do have a little concern about being totally off medication the day before because if I go three hours without the meds, I can hardly move or talk. If I sleep for six hours I am almost immobile. I try to take two pills during the night. In four hours I am almost totally off.

November 3, 2008—
Medical Planning: Deep Brain Stimulation
The Tests

1. I met with PD specialist Dr. Joseph Jankovich, Baylor Medical Clinic, to determine if I have a good reason for the surgery and to evaluate me totally off-his-pills/ on-his-pills. We were referred to Dr. Jankovich (by Dr. John Hastings) as being the closest doctor involved in PD research, which we are highly interested in. We've met with him three or four times now. I was really struggling being off my pills. I went to my appointment in a wheelchair and was reduced to a shuffle and was extremely stiff. Once I was in Dr. Jankovich's office, he watched me walk while off my pills, checked my balance, and asked me generally how I felt. Then I took my pills. He evaluated the efficacy of the PD

pills because my body will react just as positively (or not) to the DBS. I had an excellent response when on my pills. Also, my reasons were as follows, as to the surgery benefiting me in a viable way:

a.   I could expect more time between pills. I may be able to go from the current two-hour pill administrations to four to five hours. What a blessing that would be!

b.   More "up" time and less "down" time. When the pills begin wearing off and before the next dosage takes hold, sometimes there is a period of slow movement, shuffling steps, PD symptoms revealing themselves in full force. This is called "down time." The question here was: Would he make good use of more up time? Oh, my, yes! Without a doubt.

2.   We met with the surgeon who will perform the procedure. Dr. Simpson, neurosurgeon from the Methodist Hospital, spent maybe 30 minutes with us to ensure that we had all questions answered and to discuss if he thought I would be a good candidate. Again, a resounding "Yes." Dr. Simpson has now conducted 1,100 DBS surgeries and assured us that he has *never* lost a patient.

3.   Next was Dr. York, neuropsychology specialist from Baylor College of Medicine. She performed extensive psychology tests. She conducted two hours of psychology tests. She does this to ensure that any prospective DBS patient is not demented in any way. She said that patients who already have some dementia

worsen after undergoing DBS, so the doctors ensure this is not a factor. They will not perform surgery on someone who has dementia. By some miracle I passed the dementia testing!

Related Matters

If we get the call today, we would go in for surgery as soon as mid-December. It is a four- to five-hour procedure that starts around 7:00 a.m. and then I will be in the hospital through the night and if all goes well, I will be dismissed on Day Two. The second surgery is approximately ten days later, when the battery boxes are inserted—usually around the collar bone and then around the rib cage. This particular doctor said that it would be on the same side of my body. Each pack provides current either to the left or right side of the brain.

DBS is now considered a commercial [non-experimental] operation. I am opting to go for a new device that is used to implant the electrodes in the brain that is still in the research phase. By doing this, I will get the research follow-ups for free and I will get more attention than with the older device. This procedure is covered under Medicare, which I go on in December.

January 15, 2009—
Correspondence: Deep Brain Stimulation
Note To: M.

The upside for the commercial DBS system is that it has a pretty good history. Seventy percent increase in uptime hours to a total of eight and one half per day. There are many medical offices that can adjust the commercial model [that is, they can increase or decrease the voltage which should result in a corresponding increase or decrease in the amount of levodopa to the brain]. If I were to stay on the research side I would have to take many tests and many more trips to Houston to monitor the data. The trips to Houston cost $1,000 each and I can't sit on an airplane for more than an hour or I get stiff. Also, there are urination difficulties. When I have to go, I have to go.

The research is basically the same, but the doctor wants to try a different control mechanism. The commercial DBS system adjusts voltage [in other words, it can deliver varying amounts of voltage based on how it is programmed]. The new one will adjust amps. I think I need to move quickly as the pills are only effective for 1 hour 45 minutes and the time is getting shorter. I cannot go anywhere without getting the stutter steps. They see me coming and leaving with a cane and Karen holding me up at football games. I get downtime effects about twice each day. I will not just lie down and feel sorry for myself.

I am so glad I asked for a research doctor to work with, otherwise I might be months away from getting DBS. I have talked with the surgery coordinator today. We decided not to do the study, but do the current commercial DBS. I am approved for this surgery. No additional tests are required. It is a total go!

January 22, 2009—
Deep Brain Stimulation: Preparation

Well, we are down to single digits, eight days to go. The last time I counted days was in 1969 in Vietnam. It was normal for soldiers to count down from 100. I had a sergeant who slept in a bunker for the last 30 days; the mosquitoes loved him. I made it to nine and then received early out orders. I arrived home on Christmas Eve. This was the same date my dad arrived home from World War II.

I want to thank Rod MacIlvaine and the elders from Grace Community Church for praying for me and others. I am truly touched to have so many caring for me. I prayed for my surgeon, too. That is very important.

Karen and I visited with the coordinator and Dr. Richard Simpson, the surgeon. We prepared the following schedule:

- February 16—Drive to Houston: 550 miles, will need lots of breaks.

- February 18—Meetings with Dr. Simpson, Dr. Jankovich, Dr. York. Also, I believe they clamp on the metal halo with screws. I could say it, but I won't.

- February 19—Do the deed—surgery to implant the four leads. I always wanted to be bald. I will stay one night in the Methodist Hospital, Baylor University. Surgery lasts three to five hours. The longest portion is shaving my head. I am supposed to be awake during the surgery time with no pills for 12 hours. I will be a basket case. What a ride!

- February 22–26—This will be the time to place two boxes somewhere around the collar bone. It depends on whether I am ready or Dr. Simpson is ready. I think I will be ready. He can expect to replace them every two to four years. I believe if two are implanted, you can expect four years.

- March 6–9—Activate the system. It is normal for them to wait three weeks to turn it on. Seems like some folks get good results for a few weeks after surgery. I would get excited, too, if I saw four electrical leads coming directly for me.

The Houston surgeon has performed 1,100 DBS surgeries and the worst problem was a few minor infections that were treated immediately with no problems. Besides, I cannot wait to see how handsome I will be with a bald head.

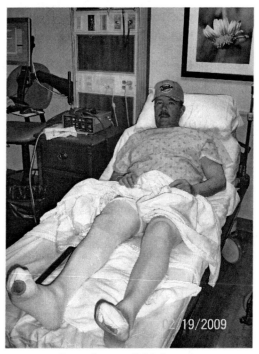

Barry Prior to DBS Surgery

January 25, 2009—
Activities/Personal Reflections

For the first time, I have real anxiety about what is going to happen to me. I will have DBS on February 19 in Houston, Texas.

- Today we celebrated Bud and Marlene's 55th wedding anniversary. A dinner at the Hotel Phillips. Very good. Attendees: Frank and Dana Jordan, Dean Horsman, Ryan Jordan, Bud and Marlene, Karen and I.

- Could not go to sleep.

- With the ongoing assault of PD, I am more concerned about safety. Because I can no longer defend me or Karen. I get anxious going to places for the first time. I would rather stay home. I worry that Karen will be upset because she wants to see and go and do new things. I do not. By the way, Karen has been great for the past three years. We have both adjusted and love each other dearly.

- I am concerned about where we will stay in Houston. It is the Hotel ZaZa. I wonder if it is in a good neighborhood or not. We talked about staying in Galveston at first, but now I wonder if it will be isolated, because I look feeble now. I am more susceptible to being attacked. This is a fact. The handicapped tag on the visor tells everyone. Three weeks between the two surgeries sounded good because I wanted to rest and watch some good family movies. I do not like violent movies. I wish I could do this DBS at home, but I cannot.

- The next three days I will be very busy. Monday, I will go to the lake from Stillwater. It is Bedlam basketball time. [This refers to a competition in the ongoing rivalry between the University of Oklahoma Sooners and the Oklahoma State University Cowboys.] We will not get home until 1:00 a.m. On Tuesday, I have a physical at 9:00 a.m. We will take Frank and Dana to the airport, attend the Real Life Real Choices meeting, attend the bid opening, and attend the technology meeting. This is too much! Just looked back at the June 28 pill schedule. It is almost identical to today. Cycle times (times between pill dosages) are down to 1 hour 50 minutes.

- So many good things have happened to me in my life.

  - Karen is super.

  - Selected the most progressive citizen of 2008.

  - Was in the top 50 [Oklahomans] of AARP.

  - We now have a dog named Chance.

  - I have three grandchildren.

  - Going south, so must stop. Cannot read my own writing.

  - I have purchased 13 cemetery plots for the family.

January 30, 2009—Pill Schedule

7:30 a.m.—one carbidopa/levodopa, one Lotrel, one Provigil, one Mirapex

9:30 a.m.—one carbidopa/levodopa, one Provigil, one amantadine

11:30 a.m.—one carbidopa/levodopa, one Mirapex

1:30 p.m.—one carbidopa/levodopa

3:30 p.m.—one carbidopa/levodopa, one Mirapex

5:30 p.m.—one carbidopa/levodopa

7:30 p.m.—one carbidopa/levodopa, one amantadine
9:30 p.m.—one carbidopa/levodopa, one Seroquel, one Sinemet CR, one Vesicare, two ex-lax
12:00 midnight—one carbidopa/levodopa
3:30 a.m.—one carbidopa/levodopa
6–6:30 a.m.—one carbidopa/levodopa

- Stopped Azilect January 26, 2009.

- Stopped Celebrex January 30, 2009.

February 12, 2009—Living with Parkinson's

I see myself as somewhat of a poster man for PD. Therefore, I will start to include information about PD in my notes. Most people look at a person with PD and feel sorry for them, with their tremors or stiffness. That is only a minor part of the problem. Seventy-five percent of people with PD have tremors; the rest of us have stiffness. *I am one of the stiffs.* Folks learn that the majority of PD people have dementia and they know there is no cure. The only truly effective drug is carbidopa/levodopa and it was made available in 1973. A little bit scary. Again, we have touched only a small portion of PD. PD attacks every muscle in your body. Did you know that PD causes 40 percent of its victims to have double vision? Because of this, I cannot put a screwdriver in the slots of the screw. And on TV all people are double—eight inches apart. In my eyes, two Rambos wipe out 1,000 bad guys.

I read an article about DBS yesterday. It stated the following:

- DBS is the only option when meds stop being effective.

- If the drugs don't help reduce things like tremors, DBS won't do it.

- DBS has a 40 percent complication rate.

February 18, 2009—
Deep Brain Stimulation: Preparation

The Hotel ZaZa is definitely top tier. Karen did a great job. During my 33-year career with lots of travel, I never was involved in a fire alarm until last night. It was a false alarm, but I got to use my training as a fire chief. I'll bet not too many of you knew I was a fire chief. I even had fire training at Texas A&M University.

We will switch from the ZaZa to a Marriott that is one block from the Methodist Hospital where the fun takes place. Another no eat, no drink, no pills after midnight. I am to be at the surgery area at 6:00 a.m. Karen gets to push me in a wheelchair because I will be unable to walk. I understand the procedure is simple:

- Shave head.

- Put on halo (it weighs 30 pounds).

- Drill two holes.

- Find brain.

- Put in wires.

Just like installing a receptacle box.

February 26, 2009—
Deep Brain Stimulation: Operation Results

Today is D+7 or D-1. It has been seven days since the first operation and one day until the next one, tomorrow. It could be D+7 because it feels like it was just yesterday and they took me into that room and placed me in that little cocoon. After tomorrow's surgery, they said I will know what it feels like to have a breast implant—two of them in fact. How lucky can a guy get! They are also supposed to hook up the wires tomorrow and will take out the staples in my head. That will be nice. When I take off my hat, with all the silver, it shines like a new sun with a bald head and aluminum spotlights. I'm sorry you all don't get a chance to see this; it will be gone by tomorrow.

After surgery, we plan to go down to Galveston for a few days and wait for the time they will actually do the programming, which will take place on March 9. I think I have mentioned to a few of you that people have received positive benefits from the device before it is even turned on. I was really interested to see how I would react to this device. I've had to cut down my medication dramatically. Otherwise, I would overdose quickly.

The doctors always say they don't understand why this happens when they run the wire by the brain cells. To me, it is pretty simple. Pretend for a minute that you are a brain cell. You are quite small, hidden in the head, protected from light and going about your business and you can over react and under react as desired. After 63 years of being my brain cell, this huge metal object comes right at you: Four of them, coming from everywhere. Wouldn't you be excited, too? I think it is like the Titanic coming down upon you if you are out in the ocean swimming. After awhile, as the brain cell gets used to the fact that this huge hunk of metal is benign, it goes back to acting the way it used to. That is when they start the programming, adjusting the voltage to make me slow down and waltz.

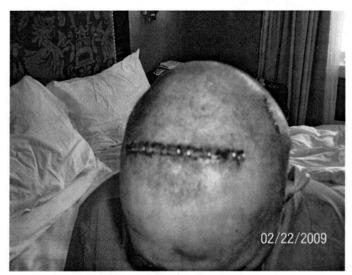

Barry's Head After DBS Surgery

March 4, 2009—Activities/Medical Condition

Things continue to improve. Karen was very successful in moving up our doctor appointments from next Monday to this Friday. We expect to leave Houston around 4:00 p.m. on Friday. The staples will be removed by Dr. Bumpus on Monday. I have a red swelling on one of my incisions. Karen is taking pictures of them and sending them to the doctor. Technology is wonderful—Wow!

We believe it is under control; taking antibiotics, looks better every day. Of course, watching the Cowboys beat K-State helped. After they cleaned OU's clocks on Sunday, I may be totally healed. I was not talking too well for a few days and Karen took over. Everything Karen said was accurate. I am doing much better now.

March 20, 2009—Activities/Operations Results

This has been an adventure, yes. Karen and I both felt God's power and love during both surgeries. Thank you and please thank all your church members for their prayers. Karen and I had no worries and I never doubted while in the waiting room that I would not be okay. Someone recently said "You must have been worried sick." Honestly, we both felt at peace about the entire situation as we felt the powers of your prayers as they embraced us in loving warmth. It took us to a higher, peaceful ground.

The healing process went nicely and I regained strength and stamina quickly. Praise God! On March 6, the power devices were turned on. In the doctor's office, we experienced immediate relief and hope. My walk went from a shuffle to not a complete stride, but a promising one. We hope that by reducing the quantity and number of times per day of my meds I will be brought up to my normal up time.

May 3, 2009—Medications/Activities

Current situation is that I am trying to find a pill combination that will give me the longest up time. I was at 1 hour 45 minutes before surgery. Today, the up times between pill dosages were 3:00, 4:00, and 5:00. Of course, I lose an hour of pretty severe down time at the end of each cycle.

Karen and I went to the Bartlesville Legends awards banquet. I had to stumble out after 3½ hours. Normally, I can only sit down for 2½ hours. After the two-hour stretch period, seems like the lack of activity reinforces the contracted muscles from PD. It seems like most people understand, but there are many who do not. I try to be as active as I can be, but I warn folks who invite us to a major event that I must be seated close to a door and there is a possibility that I might not show up. The only other option is you will sit in a corner, and I'm not ready to do that.

May 23, 2009—Parkinson's Information

We went to a PD symposium in Tulsa. One doctor was trying to make the case that DBS was a common procedure. So, he asked the audience of approximately 500. Five people raised their hands—only five. I cannot imagine why people wouldn't want to rush to the nearest surgeon. It is a unique experience to hear your skull being crushed. So you know how much is missing, they give you a handheld mirror so you can see how much is left. Not a single raised hand was shaking. There goes my humor again!

During the first reprogramming on my brain, my whole body was tingling. We were trying to eliminate the slurring and increase the right-side body muscles. One of the benefits of DBS is that it prevents you from having such low lows. It did, but for the past few days, it has also eliminated the up time. No up time yesterday, and today I have a very little from 6:30 p.m. to 9:00 p.m.

To conclude, I will pass on a few tidbits of information I gleaned from the symposium. Only 40 percent of PD patients get Alzheimer's. Are we lucky or what? PD patients do not lose their cognitive capabilities, they just think slower. I need to get slower-thinking friends. That leaves all of you out.

June 14, 2009—
Functioning Ability: Balance and Falls

Well, it has been almost four months since DBS surgery. Time sure flies when you are having fun! I promised in one of my earliest notes that my goal was to educate those who have PD and those who have friends who have PD. Many of you enjoy my dry humor, but I wanted to tell it like it is. If you see me as a wuss, so be it. So here goes.

A major side effect of PD is that you lose your sense of balance. I have been falling on a regular basis for six months now. I wish this regularity was demonstrated in other bodily functions.

When your doctor gets to know you better, he will tell you that PD will not do you in, but it will clear the way for the eventual culprits. Falls are a good example. My two falls on the slope in front of our lake house, which is a slope greater than 90 degrees, occurred as I moved from bent over to standing position; I lost my balance and fell backward. I grabbed a limb of a tree as I rolled over on the right shoulder. Something broke. The doctor had an X-ray, but could not find any tears. Well, that was about four months ago and I still cannot lift four pounds up to my waist. Of course, I cannot use this arm to catch myself when I lose my balance.

July 15, 2009—Medications Adjustment

Well, Karen and I visited Tulsa again. This is our third visit. Karen and I are taking a more proactive involvement. Not a surprise to anyone who knows us. The last reprogram was not effective. The up time was decreasing and I was falling down like those "fainting goats" you see on television. Karen and I figured out that Mirapex was causing the problem, so I ramped down, and currently I take none of this drug. We told the doctor and he was a little sad. He told us that Mirapex increased the up time of Sinemet. I told him I doubt I could survive the additional falls. The current tally was two broken ribs, a few cracked ribs, two dislocated thumbs, and some of the most beautifully colored bruises you have seen. He deferred.

July 24, 2009—
Medical Condition/Functioning Ability

First, I want to thank all of you for letting me get some things off my chest. No, this is not fun, but if I can't put some humor in the mix, I will go crazy and Karen would really have a rough job. I thank God for her every day.

Also, I appreciate the kind invitations you send to me, but I know you understand that I can only have six to eight normal hours per day, and it is a different six to eight from one day to the next. I am my own worst enemy if I don't take the pills on schedule. I am pretty good; you all know I hate details.

Well, today is going to be "pride goeth before a fall" day. Now that I think about it, I can fall before and after. I will explain how you all can help me or other PD patients.

Remember, only 25 percent of us are stiff; the other 75 percent have tremors. I really need to reduce my falls. Stopping Mirapex has helped, but I still fall. I do not get dizzy; my center of gravity goes in front of my toes and I become a gymnast. So, if you see me drop something or I look like I am going to try to bend over, please go ahead and pick it up for me. My right shoulder and my right hand cannot take any force, so I must stop the fall with my right elbow or my face. Maybe I will get one of those rugged faces and become a TV star. Maybe I will look like Lon Chaney.

My fourth programming is working okay. I have 2 hours 45 minutes between cycles. I really need that Mirapex. As I mentioned earlier, I must get better at taking my pills on time.

I take my pills on the following schedule: 7:30 a.m., 10:15 a.m., 1:00 p.m., 3:30 p.m., 6:30 p.m., and 9:15 p.m.

Valid reasons for not being on schedule include a time relationship with meals. I am supposed to take pills on an empty stomach. It is recommended that I take my pills at least one hour before eating. The levodopa transfer mechanism will preferentially process the proteins in food. So, if I have eaten a large Thanksgiving dinner, my stomach is full of turkey protein. It takes two hours to process the protein and the levadopa, with a half-life of two hours, will lose effectiveness.

Finally, my hearing continues to get worse. They tell me parts of my ears are basically dead. Amplification will not help. So if I cannot hear, saying the same thing over will not help. Spelling the words works most of the time. The worst thing is when I think I hear something and I answer what I think I heard, not what you said. So, if my answer seems out of place, help me. By the way, my hearing loss started in Vietnam. Ironically, I especially cannot hear an Asian lady at all when they talk; they are naturally quite soft-spoken. I still feel lucky to only have a hearing loss. I made it home in one piece and many were not as fortunate.

Karen and I are going on vacation beginning August 10. We are going to visit my brother and sister and Karen's daughter. We will see how I handle driving long distances. Thanks for being there for me.

August 27, 2009—Functioning Ability: Falls

This old body did not like the traveling. It was great to have so many low-key visits.

The next three weeks were involved with falling. I had three significant falls. To summarize the falls, the result of the first one was one broken rib, and the second one resulted in a torn rotator cuff. They also discovered a lot of scar tissue and arthritis. The third fall gave me a minor concussion. I never had one of those before. They can take the pizzazz out of life. Anyway, the bottom line is that surgery is required on the shoulder. The good news is that they checked my hip and it is in good shape after 16 years with no screws.

This falling stuff is starting to get me down—another good line. They continue to pop into my slow-thinking, confused head.

September 27, 2009—Hospital Stay

This is the real Barry coming to you from earth. The last two weeks have been extremely interesting. There have been five or six days in the last two weeks that I have no idea what was going on. For instance, I was at the Jane Phillips Hospital for four days and I don't remember a single thing about going, being, or leaving there.

On Wednesday of last week, they did a CT scan at the Jane Phillips Hospital and determined that I had fluid on the brain and I needed surgery. Since JP Hospital has no neurosurgeons, they transferred me to St. John's in Tulsa, where Dr. Rapake became my surgeon. They operated on me at 10:00 p.m. It lasted about an hour, and my recovery time since then has been interesting as well. Due to time constraints, I will jump over that and say that they believe that the surgery was successful.

They will be taking another CT scan tomorrow to determine if there is still bleeding into the brain from other areas. The doctor said that there is a 70 percent chance that no additional surgery will be required. And since he grew up in a town that is 50 miles from a town where I grew up, I am very optimistic as well.

I still have instances of when the brain takes over and I act in strange ways. In fact, one was yesterday morning, 1½ hours of which I have no recollection. I continue to be thankful for your kind thoughts and prayers.

I just found out that they are moving me out of neuro-ICU tonight at 6:30 p.m. to a normal room. Possibly I will be released tomorrow from St. John's and will return to Bartlesville.

October 9, 2009—Hospital Stay/
Assistive and Protective Equipment

Today I will fill in some of the details about the last two weeks. There was a five-day period when I was totally gone; I do not know where. I was at the Jane Phillips Hospital for four days and four nights and I don't remember a thing about them. I had fallen 12 times over the weekend; again, I remembered nothing of this. Karen drove me to the hospital.

Personnel at the Jane Phillips Hospital worked with me for four days trying to find out why I was falling so much. They could not find anything wrong and so they wanted to discharge me. The fact is, I had deteriorated so much in the hospital that they wanted to discharge me to a nursing home. Karen kept harping that I was a vibrant, contributing member of society "last week" and there was something they were missing. Karen said "no" to the discharge. This was not going to happen—putting me in a nursing home. Karen and I have agreed and decided we would not put one another in a full-time nursing home.

Additionally, if I would have been placed in a nursing

home without that CT scan, I wouldn't be here. Finally, they discovered that I had a subdural hematoma. If they wouldn't have found that, I may have been dead within 24 hours. They rushed me to Tulsa as they do not have a neurosurgeon in Bartlesville.

One thing that could go wrong with this type of surgery is that there is old blood within the skull. They have to remove a major portion of the skull and scrape it out. Fortunately, they did not have to do that. Melissa, my daughter, told me that she had this very bad feeling in her stomach as they wheeled me to the surgery room because she knew that I didn't know what was happening to me. It is hard to fight something of which you aren't aware.

Dr. Rapake completed the surgery in about an hour. They wheeled me back into my room. Melissa told me I looked ten years younger. The only reason I could figure I looked ten years younger was because my guardian angel was riding with me (again, thanks for those prayers). Anyway, I'm not going back into surgery to look another ten years younger. I don't want to look younger than Karen. That would make her feel bad.

I understand that the subdural hematoma will continue to be very dangerous for the rest of my life. If I fall again and hit the same spot, it could be all over. As a neurologist here in town said, "You may fall asleep and never wake up again." This is not the first time that I have faced the possibility of death. Dr. Rapake seemed disappointed that I did not respond with concern about the chance that I could die. What he wasn't aware of is the fact that there were 22 instances where I was close to dying in my life.

About a week after surgery, I was sent back to the Jane Phillips Hospital for rehabilitative therapy. I was put under extreme measures to prevent me from falling. I did not remember being told how dangerous the surgery was and how it was going to impact the rest of my life. I get it now.

So far, PD has caused these additional problems to my body and to my health: in the past three months, I've broken two ribs, dislocated two thumbs, had a concussion, and now emergency brain surgery—not to mention lots of cuts and bruises all over my body.

On the humorous side of things, I told Karen that I have become accustomed to having women in the shower with me. They watched me all the time to make sure I didn't fall. The government actually pays people to watch me pull my drawers down and pull them back up. Their story was that their watchfulness was for them to determine my mobility level.

In the six days that I was in the hospital, either at Bartlesville or Tulsa, I only had one or two hours of sleep per night. I told everyone that I needed more sleep and that sleep deprivation was becoming a reality. Fortunately, I made friends with some of the nurse's aides and they made sure that I got to talk to Dr. Zeiders, who was the head of the rehab unit in Bartlesville. He agreed that the work they were doing for me now was for PD and not for the subdural hematoma.

When I got home, I slept 12 hours the first night, 11 hours the second night, and 10 hours ever since then. I usually go to bed at 9:00 p.m. until 2:00 a.m. and work at my desk for two hours and then go back to sleep for another four hours. As I mentioned before, PD will not let me sleep for more than a few hours each time.

PD: It never stops taking. Today one of my tooth caps broke in half. The dentist told me that anesthesiologists tend to break these teeth. Today I had a root of one of these capped teeth cut out of my jaw. I wonder how many surprises I have waiting for me down my path. I have started physical therapy three times per week.

I need to prevent my falling, as any future fall could be my last. Karen is a real trooper. She has purchased and installed a chair lift for the stairway and I use it 100 percent of the time. It eliminates the opportunity for me to fall on the stairway. Also, I have just purchased a varsity grade batting helmet which I wear when appropriate (working in the yard), so that if I fall, I will be protected (my head anyway). I'm also considering buying hip pads to complete my sexy figure. Okay, the real reason is to protect my hips against contusions (black and blue bruises) and to safeguard me from breaking my hip.

It's been a rough road to travel, but I still have my head above water. Karen says I have a great attitude; I appreciate all your thoughts and prayers. Hope this report provides you with an update, some humor, and the philosophy that no matter what our life's challenges, we should never give up.

October 21, 2009—Medications/Hospital Stay

[More on the recent hospital visits:] A single night's sleep loss causes long-lasting cognitive disruptions in fruit flies comparable to PD associated dementia. The researchers found not only that a single night's sleep loss caused long-lasting obstruction in the fly's cognitive ability, but also that they are able to block this effect by feeding the flies large doses of the spice curcumin.

I was very upset with both hospitals because I was only getting one hour of sleep per night. I was definitely showing signs of sleep deprivation, but no one cared. I was told "no one sleeps well in a hospital." They gave me pain medication. It did not work. The beds were soft and the blankets were thread worn. I had not seen a doctor in the six days no matter how many times I asked. Finally, I befriended a nurse assistant who passed my request directly to the doctor. He agreed that I no longer required therapy, and I was discharged that afternoon. I slept 23 hours in the next 30 hours. I was told I was having hallucinations, so take the above with a grain of salt, but I believe them to be true.

This has been another interesting week. My new urologist has changed my medication. If you get PD, be prepared. One doctor will tell you to use all of the Sinemet you want, others say to get off of Sinemet because long-term use will cause lack of predictability of benefits and a generation of new and more severe side effects. I think someone told me that my high use of Sinemet attributed to the bleeding of the brain. My previous doctor had me up to 4,000 mg of Sinemet per day and now I take 850 mg per day. Of course, the use of 4,000 mg of Sinemet per day may be why he recommended DBS. [Use of Sinemet is favored by those who don't like the risks of DBS. DBS however, also has potentially good results. My cycle time increased from one hour 45 minutes to three hours 15 minutes and my med usage has dropped almost 50 percent. A Parkinsonian has few choices and they all have risks and rewards.]

Now, an update on the doctor who stated that I should use DBS and Stalevo: [Stalevo is levodopa, carbidopa, and entacapone] The doctor said to take only five of the 150 mg Stalevo pills per day plus one 100 mg dose at night. This means I will have some low times several times per day. This puts me at 850 mg per day. So you will see me stutter stepping more often out in public than you did before.

October 22, 2009—Medications Management

1. The cost of Stalevo, 100 mg and 150 mg, was $200 per month.

2. I'm taking one tablet of Provigil twice a day (in the morning) instead of half a tablet which I was doing for a few days (I was trying to cut back and it wasn't working).

3. With 150 mg of Stalevo I get very active.

4. When I go to rehab, 150 is not sufficient. I always use carbidopa/levodopa at a higher rate when I exercise. Because of physical exertion, it appears that I use up more meds than normal. Am I allowed to make adjustments for this with Stalevo? Suggest 100 mg before rehab and 100 mg after.

5. I've tried not to take Stalevo 100 mg when I go to sleep. I wake up six hours later and cannot go to sleep. I suggest I don't take that pill until the middle of the night (around 4:00 a.m.), which makes it six hours after the last 150 mg.

6. Then I take Stalevo 150 mg at 11:00 p.m. It appears that Clonazepam is effective in allowing me to sleep without nightmares. I still wake up three times per night to relieve myself; without any sleep aids, I was awakening 9–10 times per night. Of course, I'm no longer taking Seroquel as in the past. Clonazepam

has effectively replaced the Seroquel as a nighttime sleep aid.

October 23, 2009—
Activities/Medications Management

My driver's license has been pulled by the state of Oklahoma because I have advanced PD. No real reason was given except I might not be able to respond correctly to extreme situations. My cognitive thinking was tested and I got every exercise correct and I am smart enough to be extremely careful when my physical skills are being restricted. This will limit my capability to maintain my activities, and if I just hang out at home, I will go crazy. I can't wait until spring so I can get outside. Of course, I will wear my major league batting helmet, so if I fall and hit my head, I will be okay.

I must admit that when I changed drugs the past nine years, I fell asleep while driving, made some poor decisions, but learned how to handle this. I mention this because a person who has PD should know of the possibility that freedom of movement may be taken away.

The doctors are split on how much levodopa a person should take. I was up to greater than 3,000 mg per day and my doctor said I should stay below 850 mg. In fact, some doctors believe my high usage of Sinemet [containing levodopa and carbidopa] caused many falls, which resulted in minor long-term hemorrhaging of the brain. This ended up being a subdural hematoma.

- DBS is most effective where the swing between on/off is extreme—really "high highs" and really "low lows." When this is the case, the highs are extended. I am currently at 1 hour 45 minutes, nine times per day. For about half of my lows, I must go lie down immediately. Seventy-five percent of the folks who have DBS get an additional seven hours per day of high-quality "on" time.

- I told the doctor that the Stalevo pills and Apokyn injectable gave inconsistent results. He said, "That's what happens in the fifth stage." The good news was that I was the worst physically that I would get. I cannot walk very far. I cannot stand erect very long. When I am at the really low-lows I cannot think, write my name, pickup a pencil or drive my electric cart. It will be tough on me because I am not a laid-back guy and I must learn to live with my handicap. I will endeavor to persevere.

- If I remember correctly, the levodopa is absorbed in the small intestine and when you are on Sinemet, you are expected to take pills on an empty stomach or take the pills one hour before eating or two hours after eating. On a three-hour cycle, like mine, that is difficult. Also, the transport mechanism will preferentially transport protein, so a low protein diet is recommended with Stalevo which has entacapone in addition to levodopa. Carbidopa has no such restrictions and entacapone has nothing to do with the absorption of levodopa. The last bit of info required to understand my proposal is the half-life of levodopa, four hours. This means it is at 100 percent strength at hour 1, 50 percent at hour 2, 25 percent at hour 8, 12.5 percent at 12. Now, remember that one of the pill's side effects is chronic constipation.

- If you have chronic constipation, the levodopa will time out in your stomach and very little will be absorbed by the small intestine. I usually experience three to four days of constipation and I get real fatigued and sleep for two hours, then I feel great. Using backward-looking logic: My cousin visited us from West Virginia; it was a great two days. On the way to the airport, we had Mexican food. I realized I took the pills a few hours before eating. It had cheese on it; it was good, but isn't cheese protein? I did a double-whammy to myself and paid for it for the next eight hours—like I had gone off the drugs cold-turkey.

• Apokyn injection was prescribed. A 90-day supply costs $20,000. I was blown away. I used very little because the results were very different. Sometimes I would take it and it would work great because it would extend the pills to a six-hour cycle and other times it would make me very drowsy and I would go to sleep immediately. I have made the assumption that Apokyn will extend whatever mood I'm in. It will not make the lows go away. I plan to try to take it when I am normal. I must be careful because sometimes it gets me high. That is not good either.

As for drug status, the injectable drug Apokyn continues to be beneficial. It seems to extend the effectiveness of the pills to four hours. I had a little trouble and I remembered I left the bag in the truck one night and the liquid froze. It is not supposed to do that. I threw the bottle out, put in a fresh one, and no problem so far. At our last office visit, he turned up the boxes one notch each [on the DBS system]. Maybe this will give me extra time.

November 4, 2009—Correspondence
Update To: Doctor

1. When I take my second set of pills around 11:00 a.m., I get very tired and dizzy.

2. When I do rehab or yard work, the cycles are shorter by 15–30 minutes.

3. Stalevo start-up time is longer than Sinemet. Sinemet would start within 30–40 minutes. Stalevo takes 1 hour 30 minutes before I feel the effect of the pill.

4. I have endured longer underdose symptoms in order to sleep better.

5. I start feeling bubbles [It feels like bubbles popping in my knee] after 2 hours 45 minutes, which usually means the pills are losing their effectiveness.

6. I have never had entacapone. It seems to be a prerequisite before taking Stalevo in the documentation I have read.

7. Clonazepam continues to work well as my Seroquel replacement.

8. I have had only three high periods in the last two weeks.

9. In the past two weeks, I have used five Stalevo 150s and one Stalevo 100 per day.

10. The effectiveness of Stalevo 150 starts wearing off after about 2 hours 45 minutes. I went to 3:15 at your request; however, it was not a pleasant journey. If I go to 3:30, the lows get lower.

November 4, 2009—
Parkinson's Information/Emergency Room Visit

Ready for stimulating research? Well, here it comes.

In fertility reproduction studies for carbidopa/levodopa, no effects on fertility were found in rats receiving dosages of approximately two times the maximum dose. It is up to others less experienced than I to comment on the test animals that were selected.

Since the Vietnam War, Steve Fiscus was convinced there was a link between Agent Orange and PD. Due in large part to a study published by the Institute of Medicine, the VA Department has imposed new rules recognizing the link between Agent Orange and PD.

Having personally been exposed to Agent Orange during combat operations, I have proposed the following questions to myself. Would I prefer to be shot by someone hiding in the vegetation or die 30 years later as a victim of Agent Orange? I have my answer. What is yours?

Did you know that the average person generates 1.5 liters of saliva per day? We Parkinsonians actually generate less than the average person. That thing hanging from our chin shows how efficient we are. My wife asks me, "Don't you feel that?" Of course we don't. It is like a wart, only better looking. The lower classes call it slobber; to us, it is saliva. It also helps us with wind direction and speed.

As for me, I am still paying for the three-piece appliance that was probably broken by a sleep doctor [anesthesiologist]. The dentist charged $625 to take out two roots. I know why poor folks have such pretty smiles.

As I have switched to Stalevo, my down time has increased,

not decreased. Anyway, I sure hope this works, because the last four weeks have not been fun.

I thought I had better explain the following very quickly so you get it straight from the horse's mouth. Yesterday, Melissa and I went downtown. As we walked to the parking lot, I tripped on a sewer cleanout that was sticking out of the ground about two inches. Many of you are old enough to remember Dogpatch in the comic strips. There was a fellow who walked around with a cloud over his head. His name was Joe. The only luck he ever had was bad luck. I'm starting to feel that way. Anyway, I fell and could not get up. As it turns out, my left shoulder came out of the socket. Everyone was very polite and helpful. As I got up on the X-ray table, I heard something pop. I told the doctor he could take another X-ray. The shoulder had snapped back into place.

Many of you have offered to help me. I'm going to take you up on your offer. Now that I have two disabled arms, I need some muscle and I don't want to work my caregiver too much. Here goes. I have been making a major effort to move things out of the house. Jane Phillips' fifth grade class is having a garage sale. I have many suitcases, a baby bed, games, etc., that must be taken to Jane Phillips or Mary Martha Outreach.

November 12, 2009—
Parkinson's Information/Medications

Agent Orange update: It was pointed out to me that *Kiplinger's Retirement Report* said that PD had been added to the list of medical conditions that are presumed to have been caused by Agent Orange. Therefore, monthly disability payments will be paid upon evidence of service in Vietnam plus the diagnosis of PD.

Another bubble has burst. I thought I was just a wild and crazy guy. [A major medical study was completed on the relationship between certain Parkinson's drugs and impulse control disorders.] Some individuals develop behaviors that can be described as compulsive or obsessive. Now, I have an excuse for doing crazy things. These behaviors include gambling, overeating, overdrinking, shopping, and sex. Gambling and sex are the most common. Nope, I wasn't in that study. Were any of you?

They started me on another new drug: Apokyn. It was approved in Europe in 1994. Our FDA approved it in 2004 with requirements. It is injectable and a nurse came to our house from Joplin. The purpose is to improve the down time. Ten to twenty minutes after I inject, I feel better and sometimes I go for four hours before my next pill. Also, I discovered that one of my DBS boxes had shut down. This affected my three-hour cycle times from pills only, but did not seem to impact the injections.

November 28, 2009—
Activities/Parkinson's Information

I hope you had a great Thanksgiving. I was invited to the Horsman home and the food was great—almost as good as the conversation. On Tuesday, December 15, I will have my right ruptured shoulder operated on (this is the fifteenth time that I have had surgery). I must like anesthesia. It won't be the last, as the left shoulder is next. Anyway, my personal request is that I would like to talk to someone who has had the same or similar surgery. I am really interested in knowing how to sleep and get in and out of bed. The surgeon asked me if I was healthy enough to have this surgery. I told him I wasn't getting any better; this is as good as it gets.

Research News

I must give credit where credit is due. Most of my comments in this regard are gleaned from the National PD Foundation. Of course, I add the personal touch, which probably has no basis in research, but is definitely true. My thoughts are based on personal experiences, not statistics. Once I had a job at R&D. I didn't understand what these chemists were talking about. But once again, I endeavor to persevere. Remember who said that? Anyway, I kept going to research meetings, and one day the light bulb went on. Then I understood how catalysis worked to make plastics. I was so proud of myself. So, I stayed in for the next presentation. I listened and became confused. When the presenter was finished, I turned to the person next to me and asked, "If I understood the last two presentations, they said the exact opposite." He said, "You are correct." Those were the last research presentations I attended.

I find PD is the same. Every time I change doctors, I have totally changed my medications. I have drawers full of old pills. To be specific, to get my DBS system, I spent seven hours on the surgery table, was billed over $200,000, and some doctors said I should turn it off. I was taking approximately 3,000 mg per day of levodopa. Some of the literature says 600 mg should be max. Some believe that 3,000 mg contributed to my falling, which eventually resulted in my subdural hematoma.

Now I have been on an injectable drug called Apokyn. It is supposed to improve the down cycles of PD. It actually seems to work. It lasts one hour and I am supposed to use a maximum of five per day. I reached about one per day, but it seems to work. I just wonder how people will react when I "shoot up" in the movie theater.

More Research: Do You Really Want to Know??

There are precursors to PD. I mentioned once before that loss of smell is one. I lost my capability to smell in 1967. I attributed it to where I worked. The chemicals involved included sulfuric acid fumes, fatty acid fumes, ammonia, hydrogen sulfide, caustic, and the big daddy, sulfur trioxide. I could not smell baby diapers or the men's rooms in Johnstone Park. Both pluses. But, I also could not smell my wife's perfume or fresh-baked apple pie. Real negatives. In fact, as I write this, I remember that Proctor and Gamble gave me a smelling test. I got 10 right out of 100. The Parkinson's Disease Association risk study believes loss of smell is a common first symptom in people with PD.

There is more evidence that hereditary factors in PD are a major concern. The Parkinson's Disease Foundation has partnered with a genetic company called 23andMe. For $25, they will test your saliva (or is it slobber). We have been there already.

To end on a positive note, I want to thank the HR Department of ConocoPhillips. With all my bills, I looked them over; I found over $3,500 that they wanted to pay. I disagreed and HR stood by me and I am very appreciative.

December 26, 2009—
Parkinson's Research/Caregiving

1. To an amateur like myself, some complex things look difficult, but they are truly simple. Do you remember my "Do you really want to know" segment? The results of research have been and are currently more effective

at slowing down the progress of PD at an early stage. The loss of smell can occur at least 30 years before you experience the real thing. Treating PD early will add to the quality and quantity of your life.

2. There is genetic research that has identified five genes that are linked to PD. The first study was of ethnic Japanese. The second study looked at Europeans. It was found that variants of PARK16, SNAC and LRRK2 carry risks of PD in both Japanese and Europeans, while variants of BST1 and MAPT were population specific.

3. A chemical found in green tea (EGCG) and a variety of protein structures can prevent and destroy amyloids, which are key in the development of disorders such as Alzheimer's and PD. You can purchase EGCG at a health food store.

The new injectable drug, Apokyn, does give me relief during the down time. Not as good as touted, but definitely an improvement. The drug is non-addictive and does not lose its effectiveness.

I have been giving a lot of thought lately to the change in relationship that happens when one person of a couple has PD and the other is the caregiver. Both lives are changed dramatically. I would like for all of you to join the conversation.

December 26, 2009—Correspondence
From: A Friend

My dad had PD for many years. It was eventually diagnosed as Lewy body disease, but it presented much like

PD. One thing a neurologist told us that really helped my brother and I in dealing with our dad. He said the patient believes he is sending the signals even though he shows no evidence physically of doing the desired act.

I might tell Pop to lift his foot a couple of inches off the floor so I could put his shoe on his foot. He would look at me like "How much higher do you want it?" He would still be pushing his foot against the floor. It was like he was a sassy two-year-old and very frustrating. When we realized that he was trying, that helped our attitude. Sometimes he would look like he was totally ignoring our requests.

The explanation was something like "the motivational nerves were as disconnected as the emotion nerves" so the brain thought he was cooperative even though he showed no signs of it. I shared this with a friend whose mother had PD, and she just burst into tears. She said her sister was getting so frustrated with their mom, but that insight would be tremendously helpful.

December 26, 2009—Correspondence
From: My Cousin

You keep being that boxer and never give up. The only thing I wish you would give up for the safety of everyone on the road is your driver's license. It is not easy to lose that kind of independence, but this time you should think of others whom you might kill or injure on the road.

My mother gave up everything to take care of daddy—especially when he moved into the last couple of years of PD as an invalid. She literally gave up everything: all her club activities, church, doing things with friends, everything. She wouldn't even leave him when I visited so we could go and have lunch together. Dad had an aide, and of course, home nursing care, a barber who came to the house, and so on. But, mother was always there for him. She wouldn't allow anyone to touch his colostomy area, because she was afraid they wouldn't wash it properly and she was meticulous about every aspect of his care. She did this for 15 years.

Because I witnessed what my mother had gone through, I wanted to find a balance, taking good care of my husband while keeping as much normalcy as possible. I still gave up a lot to be there for him. Every weekend I would drive to Baltimore, Friday night, stay with him and come home Sunday afternoon, go to work and then do it all over again. There wasn't time for extras. Friends came and went both at the hospital and when he came home; we always had friends interacting with us, which was wonderful. We didn't feel isolated. I went home for lunch every day (and still do) whether he had an aide there or not. He was on the feeding tube for six months so movement was definitely restricted. He was very aware of the stress I was going through and was very mindful of his requests. In fact, I was so stressed out that I got Bell's palsy. My face was badly distorted and I looked that I had a stroke. Every time I took him to the doctor, they thought I was the patient. Four months later, I recovered 95 percent.

You can't make decisions for your wife. She knew what she was getting into and if she wasn't willing to be a part of all of this, she wouldn't have married you. She loves you in all things. She is doing these things for you is out of love and because she wants to. Otherwise, she would be gone. I suggest you eliminate some of her stress by giving up the driver's license.

January 9, 2010—Correspondence
To Doctor: Drug Status

1. Provigil—We ordered 180 with three refills. Someone decided there was a quantity limit and 180 exceeded that figure. I asked for a quantity review. They agreed to the two pills per day, but we must submit a new prescription for 180 with three refills.

2. I've consistently had constipation problems. I found a package of pills: Amitiza. According to the Internet, they are approved for chronic constipation. If you agree, I will take two per day as recommended, and if they work, maybe you can provide a prescription.

3. Apokyn—I rarely use more than one per day and I believe I am not taking advantage of this shot. I still have much difficulty getting started in the morning. After two sets of pills I am stiff. Since I only take five Stalevo 150s per day, this means I will have more down time.

4. If I take the first two sets of pills with an Apokyn injection between them, many times I get four or more hours of up time on the rest of the day's pills. There seems to be a residual effect of the Apokyn. I would like to take Apokyn first thing in the morning, thereby not having so much down time. I will stay at five 150s per day, however, there are times when I take an injection and I get very dizzy and tired and usually go to sleep for an hour. Your thoughts, please. I only take .16 ml per injection and it was recommended that I take .2 to .4 ml.

January 22, 2010—
Medical Condition/Functional Ability: Falls

1. I have faithfully used the mobile chair to get to the second floor—except for two times. Karen and I were late for some meeting and I forgot my wallet, so I bypassed the chair. What could go wrong? As I came back down and got to the bottom, my bifocals mixed up the elevation of the bottom two steps. I missed the real step, fell fairly hard. This was one for my stupidity.

2. The next fall was in an alley freshly asphalted. Instead of walking in a rough field, I chose the alley where there was a sewer cap sticking up two inches, painted flat black. I did not see it. I tripped and dislocated my left shoulder. I was upset because I was trying to be careful, but bad things happened anyway. I did not hit my head.

3. I was standing in the yard and all of the sudden both feet went out from under me. I did not hit my head, but I was being careful. There was a thin layer of ice under the thin layer of snow.

4. At a recent night meeting, I was walking to my car with my cane. There was no lighting. There were two elevation changes from the sidewalk to the street. I tripped but did not fall. When I returned to the meeting, I was very careful. I could not see, everything was black or grey. I could not distinguish the elevation changes. I tripped again and fell hard. I did not strike my head, but nighttime depth perception seems to be a problem. This was January 13, 2010.

5. Karen and I were at Stillwater the other night. After the game, we headed to our vehicle. This was the first time I had parked in this particular parking lot. They had laid many concrete parking blocks everywhere so I was very careful. I spied a couple of blocks and made sure I missed them, but there was one I did not see and it got me. I fell forward and did hit the right front of my head. Again, a depth perception problem. Why didn't I have these falls before? This was January 20, 2010.

6. Sometimes I think I am just being tested. The falls didn't work, so now my PSA (prostate-specific antigen) count is rising. It has always been 1.0 or less. When I took a complete physical recommended by Medicare, my PSA count was 2.2. Dr. Bumpus suggested I start a history of PSA tests. Two weeks ago, I had one. It was 3.9. So that required an appointment with a urologist. I am starting to get tired of this body breaking down. The urologist, Dr. Peaster, said everything felt okay. I go back in four months.

7. Some good news. My cycles used to be 2 hours 45 minutes at a time, now they are extending to 4:25 to 5:00. It could be any of the following:

   a. The power to my internal boxes has been increased slightly.

   b. We added amantadine to my pill menu.

   c. I have the Apokyn injection, which addresses the low end of the cycle.

The Apokyn works well about 60 percent of the time and the rest of the time it is lousy.

On the other health news, I took large quantities of selenium, vitamin D, and flaxseed oil. My PSA went from 4.11 to 3.04 in one month. Also, the PSA test has a record of 50 percent false positives. In addition, the VA identified that I had a vitamin B12 deficiency. I am taking B12 shots once per week. No wonder I was so tired. Research just verified that vitamin D was good for PD.

February 2010—
Personal Reflections As of This Month

I was thinking about being wheelchair bound. I think I finally understood someone would have to clean me, feed me, etc. In effect, ruining two lives, which I pray doesn't happen. I believe I only ask God to guide me in doing the right thing. When He took Mom and Dad, I understood. I never understood why He took Kris—only if it was for her reward. When I was in combat, I asked for guidance in making the right decision and to not let me be a coward. Now I ask that He not let me ruin Karen's life.

This caused me to think of a letter I received from my cousin, Virginia. Her father, my Uncle Lloyd, had PD. His wife, Dani, short for Danielle, took care of him 24 hours per day. I was getting much guidance about marrying so early after Kris' passing. I won't go into that now, but Virginia asked me if Karen and I knew what we were getting into. We thought we did, but now we know we truly didn't. I feel so bad for Uncle Lloyd because he had Sinemet for only the last 14 years. Before 1973, there were no drugs to help.

I think Karen and I both realized the task before us, and we will give it our best shot. I pray to God: Please take me quick, Karen deserves a better life. My life will change; I realized today that if I went to church and I froze up, I could not bear to be carried from the room not being able to walk. We want to have a motor chair to take with us to Branson, Missouri, on May 2. Also, we will start to remodel the downstairs for a master bedroom. We have a rental electric cart now. Karen likes to take walks and with the cart I can outdistance her!

Please keep us in your prayers; you only need to know that we will fight the good fight.

We will also start looking for a wheelchair-accessible van.

March 1, 2010—
Parkinson's Information/Personal Reflections

First the good news. I have not fallen since January 20, or put another way, I have been successful at standing up for 40 days straight. In evolution that is fantastic. I feel like a frog. However ("however" is like "but," foreshadowing a negative twist), I have a very difficult time getting out of bed. In fact, without Karen's help, I could not get out. I need help with getting shirts and jackets on and off as well, so if you see me struggling, your help would be appreciated.

This update will have a different, more somber tone—so fair warning. My brain was activated by several conversations.

- With advances in genetics, I was asked if my daughters would like to know if they were going to get PD. Some people want to know; others do not. I have signed up for the research and will let you know if my genes were the problem. The bigger question is this: Does the person want to know that they will probably have a debilitating disease that attacks your whole body and you have 40 percent chance of losing your mind as well (i.e., Alzheimer's)? What good would it do to know for 30–40 years that you will meet Mr. P and you will lose? There is a plus, though. Some doctors believe if they start treatment early, they will delay the progress of the disease. Would I like to be in this feeble position for 25 years instead of 15?

- A friend asked me if I would talk to his sister who had just been diagnosed with PD, as she wanted to know what was waiting for her. Of course, I said, "Yes." That is the purpose of this diary—to let PD folks know what to expect and to educate the lucky ones who are PD-free to understand and be gracious to those who have it.

- I was looking at my personal notes written when I lost my mother, my father, and my mother-in-law in 13 weeks and then lost my wife less than a year later. I was a wreck and wrote about my deep remorse. I am not as strong as some believe. Anyway, I thought of my father, who I am convinced had PD. He suffered with back pain, shakes, slobbers, slurred speech, etc. I see myself sitting like he sat, talking fast and soft. They gave him a pill the night before his surgery, and the shakes went away. His speech was almost perfect. I think of his many years of suffering with no medication.

- I had an uncle who had PD. He passed on in 1987. He had married a wonderful woman. She quit all of her personal activities to take care of him. This makes me think of my wife. I don't want to ruin another person's life. Mine should be sufficient. When Karen and I were dating and were becoming more than just friends, I told her I had

PD and maybe we should just cool it. Since I know her better now, I suspect she got out her computer that night and knew more about PD by the next morning than most doctors. Anyway, she is quite strong-willed—some might stay stubborn—and said she would stand by her man. It still concerns me that she will sacrifice so much for this beat-up old body. To summarize, I don't want to be an invalid; I don't want to ruin another person's life. A terrible consequence is that it affects more than the person who is ill. It impacts all who care about the person as well. There is more research being directed at the impact on caregivers.

- The doctors are split on how much levodopa a person should take. I was up to greater than 3,000 mg per day and my current doctors say I should stay below 850. In fact, some doctors believe my high usage of Sinemet allowed minor long-term hemorrhaging of the brain which resulted in the subdural hematoma. With time, the hemorrhaging was so severe that a one-inch thick section of my skull was filled with blood, resulting in the brain being compressed into 90 percent of the space required. The doctors had warned my daughter that there was a good chance that I would be different when I woke up. But no such luck. The same old Barry remains. People are very kind and tell me how good I look and that my walking is really good. Now keep those compliments coming, but you don't see me in my bad times.

- Usually I can adjust the pills so I can act like a normal person for three to four hours. But if an activity takes longer, such as an eight-hour trip to the state capital, I cannot do that. I definitely need someplace to lie down.

Sitting does not work either. So when Karen and I go to Stillwater for a basketball game, I am quite stiff after sitting for two hours; a five-minute walk does not help. So we get a hotel room to refresh ourselves and we head to Bartlesville the next morning. Thus, I only schedule four hours of meetings per day, i.e., taking my medication the same time each day each day, and hope I can adjust. I cannot get up at 6:00 a.m. to attend an early breakfast one day without suffering the next several days.

Now, this is for those of us who like big words that impress and confuse others. Get ready. In this study, the transplanted embryonic neurons migrated and integrated into the correct neural circuitry of the striatum, matured into so-called GABAergic inhibitory interneurons, and dampened the overexcitation in the region. I know this is really getting me excited! The rats had improved motor function, as seen in their balance, speed, and the length of stride during walking.

The results, the scientists say, demonstrated that the transplanted cells, known as embryonic medial ganglionic eminence (MGE) cells can very precisely modify the balance of excitation and inhibition in neural circuits to influence behavior. As overactive neural circuits are associated with other neurodegenerative diseases—a result of nonfunctioning or missing cells or abnormal synaptic transmission—the finding may have broad implications.

Okay, okay, I promise no more today. Spell check just had a heart attack.

April 4, 2010—Correspondence
From: Virginia

Every time I get an update on you, my heart sinks then rises. I go from despair to pure admiration of you. The trials and tribulations you endure with PD are beyond your endurance, and yet, here you are, the amazing Barry going on with the next step, the next experiment. You are an incredible individual and my dearest cousin.

Peter (Virginia's brother) stayed mobile and gained more independence with his scooter chair. He had a trailer specially made for the back of his Fiat to transport his chair. The cart was as big as his car. He could take himself all over the place. It was easier for mother because she didn't have to push and pull a wheelchair as she did with daddy.

My darling cousin, my heart is just breaking about all you have been through and what is left for you to endure. Karen will be by your side and that will make it easier for you. At this point, don't dwell on how you might be holding her back. She has your love to keep her going. Mother never wavered and Karen won't either. You are going to have to keep communicating always and always know that you can enjoy each other as long as possible. You are my only link to my family—past and present. You are the only one who knew them all.

April 4, 2010—
Activities/Parkinson's Information

I hope everyone had a happy Easter. Karen and I just relaxed and thanked the Lord for watching over us. We were planning on heading to Branson to celebrate our fifth anniversary, but I was not well enough to go so we delayed our departure. The following articles come from the Northwest Parkinson's Disease Foundation:

1. Additional survey results show that the first symptom most patients notice is tremor (70 percent) followed by general stiffness (39 percent), loss of smell (16 percent). Furthermore, respondents report that the highest concern is how the PD will progress, followed by worry over career and finances. The highest concern is how their PD will progress. Fortunately, I am retired and was lucky with investments. Last year, my drugs cost $32,000. My portion was $6,000, but as you might recall, I was frustrated with doctors not being forthright in telling me what the future held for me. A standard answer was this: "Something else will get you first" That is why I started this epistle. I just looked, and I started this dialog December 18, 2008. Time flies when you are having fun.

2. A PD vaccine is being tested. Researchers say the vaccine would not cure PD, but would halt its progression. For slow learners like me, that means it will not get worse.

I passed several milestones since we last met! I have not fallen since our last discussion. That is 80 days fall-free, but I shuffle more. I believe this is due to my reduced medication. I have asked the doctor to increase my devices one notch each, but he has refused. There is only one neurologist in town, so ???. To be answered later.

I used an electric cart in Wal-Mart the other day. It was fun. To tell the rest of the story, for the first time, I basically froze up and could not move. Fortunately, Karen was with me and she asked if she went for a cart, would I use it. She must think I am stubborn! I told her this was a major decision. I said, "Yes." Now we are looking at purchasing one. If you have any words of wisdom, let me know.

As I mentioned earlier, some neurologists don't believe in DBS; others do. After letting them drill two holes in my head and implant two devices in my chest (thank goodness for Medicare) this doctor does not believe in increasing my DBS. He grins and I get to bear it. The Mayo Clinic is supposed to be the best hospital in this area and a clinic in Washington State has a good reputation. We will pick one before we give up on this option.

I finally read an article on how PD wins the war. You become wheelchair bound. Also, I read once that PD affects your diaphragm as well. So, it is time to begin preparation for immobility. We are already looking at power chairs and thinking of how to convert the downstairs living room into a bedroom. That will give us five bedrooms.

I still must have both shoulders operated on. I can't figure out how I am going to sleep and get out of bed without using my arms and shoulders. All advice is appreciated. Enough for now. Have a wonderful life.

April 25, 2010—Functioning Ability

First, the good news. I have not fallen in the last seven weeks. Most of this is due to the fact that it is pretty difficult to fall out of a wheelchair, but give me time. Also, I now accept the fact that I cannot take two steps without falling. I have fallen enough. To summarize for new readers, in the past year, my falls have resulted in the following: three broken ribs, two torn rotator cuffs (so bad they cannot be surgically repaired), two broken thumbs, a brain hemorrhage which required high risk emergency surgery, a major hallucination (in this hallucination I was to be sacrificed to the gods), and two puncture wounds requiring a total of 32 stitches. Each new doctor has their nurse get the historical data. Somewhere in this recount of the good old days, I ask the nurse, "Is that enough or do you need more?"

April 25, 2010—Activities/Functioning Ability

I believe this will be a challenging time for Karen and me. Having two bad shoulders and PD in both legs is like being on roller skates with only one arm at 20 percent strength. I rarely walk between rooms without calling for Karen. The stutter step puts me out of control and neither arm will support the weight. I must fall on my nose or elbows. That is not easy. So, I am becoming wheelchair bound.

We went to Branson to celebrate our fifth wedding anniversary and I rode an electric scooter all day. I didn't run into a single person. Guess I can still drive. We spent two days at Branson. We toured the Titanic exhibit, played miniature golf, and toured a condo with no sales pressure. I was surprised. At Silver Dollar City, we did the normal things: eat, listen to a trio from South America, we enjoyed ourselves.

My nephew Ryan graduated from Oklahoma State University this week with a bachelor's degree in geology. We drove to Stillwater for his graduation.

May 14, 2010—
Shoulder Surgery/Personal Reflections

The following is rather sobering, but I believe it is accurate. Much has happened during the past three weeks. Here is my medical status. My doctor thought I may have congestive heart failure, but after a $1,600 test, they decided my heart was A-okay. It's been through a lot so I'm not surprised.

The rise in my PSA count did not get my urologist excited. I will get another PSA test in June and we will look at it again.

I ended my "no fall" record of 90+ days. I was walking in bright sunlight in a parking lot and one of the slabs had risen about an inch. I went down with a thud. I learned two things: 1) Stay out of parking lots, and 2) People with PD lose depth perception. I had two bruised ribs.

I had my left shoulder surgically worked on last Tuesday. The anesthesiologist went out of her way to be certain I understood that post-surgery could be a very painful time. She was right. Glad I only have two shoulders. My BP was 135/75, so I guess I didn't get too upset. My surgeon has 35 years of experience and he told me that it was the most damaged shoulder he had seen. Cocky me, I said that maybe that is why it hurt and would I get some kind of trophy? He was pretty sharp when he told me that my right shoulder was just as bad. The good news: he was pleased with the surgery results, and the patient is still alive.

Today I may have finally accepted my fate. Karen has been quite sullen the past few days. I asked her why. It is absolutely amazing how we constantly think about the same thing at the same time though it is totally random with no link or logic. With some prodding, she said she was reading a book about the final stage of PD. In particular, one case she mentioned was where the person could only open his eyelids after five minutes of massage.

September 25, 2010—Correspondence
Update To: Doctor

1. The Sanctura was replaced with its generic, trospium, by the Veterans Administration. Do you agree? Both the Sanctura and the generic are not effective with the urgency and incontinence. What do you recommend I do? This is becoming a major problem.

2. My drug plan has told me they will replace Azilect with rasagiline. Do you agree?

3. I am working with the Veterans Administration on Agent Orange and PD. Also, we are working on hearing loss, an electric scooter and lift, my potential prostate cancer, cost of drugs, etc. What a tremendous secret they are. They fill prescriptions at $8 per month. I have several that cost me $500 per month outside the VA system. They have made substitutions:

    a. Trospium for Sanctura

    b. Rasagiline for Azilect

    c. Amlodipine besylate and enalapril maleate for Lotrel

    d. Amantadine HCL for amandatine

    e. And finally, etodolac for Celebrex

4. I have finished using the Requip 2 mg. No bad side effects. I have many 5 mg Requip from a previous doctor. Can I take two of these 5 mg per day?

5. To give you the full picture, the VA discovered that I had a B12 deficiency. Imagine PD and insufficient

B12. I am taking 1 ml injection of cyanocobalamin every two weeks.

6.   Also, in regard to my PSA testing, I have been taking selenium, vitamin B, flaxseed oil. When the VA did the testing, my number was 3.04. This is down more than 1.0 point in one month. I should get another PSA number and percent-free next week. Before taking the vitamins and minerals, I had a 4.11 PSA.

October 4, 2010—
Veteran's Administration Benefits

My relationship with the VA so far has been excellent. They checked my ears and gave me a new set of hearing aids that they say go on the market for $5,000 each. They have given me a new electric chair for $3,800 and a lift to put the chair in the back of my Tahoe. It is my understanding that the VA will supply prescription drugs for $10 for a 30-day prescription. Currently, I have prescriptions that cost in excess of $500 per month. I really believe that the VA is one of the best-kept secrets of our federal government.

The main reason I went to the VA was to get on a list of people who were exposed to Agent Orange and have since developed PD. The legislation has moved slowly through Congress, but it is my understanding that legislation is on the Hill or will be there shortly. When this legislation is signed an individual will receive 100 percent disability, which is approximately $2,750 per month, and all drug costs will be covered as a federal expense.

On the medical front, my PSA checked out by the laboratory at JP hospital gave me a number of 4.0 and a percent-free of 20, which is 2 points higher than last time. This is good. The doctor is very pleased with the results. I have been scheduled back in six months. I told them I was taking vitamin D, selenium, and flaxseed oil. He was very happy that we were doing that. This takes a lot off my mind. Since the last status report I had one minor fall into the fish pond: At least I got a new cell phone. Karen is very forward thinking and got insurance, but I have to keep this one for the next four years. I have never had a new cell phone, hearing aid, or cane that lasted that long.

April 11, 2011—Parkinson's Information

It has been a while, but I have been busy and I have passed a few major points. I promised to be up front and I will endeavor to keep that commitment. First, I finally found a book that lists stages of Parkinson's. They are as follows:

Stage 0   No signs of the disease

Stage 1   Unilateral disease—affects one side of the body

Stage 1.5   Unilateral and axial (neck and back)

Stage 2   Mild bilateral disease without impairment of balance

Stage 2.5   Mild bilateral disease with some impairment of balance

Stage 3   Mild to moderate with balance bilateral disease with some difficulty with balance still physically independent

Stage 4   Moderate to severe bilateral disease with marked disability (needs help with most major tasks such as dressing, bathing and eating). Still able to walk without a person assisting, but may need a cane or a walker.

(Hold on and be patient, I am next.)

Stage 5   Advanced disease. Wheelchair bound or bedridden unless fully aided by another person.

The doctors freely talk about my advanced PD. My current doctor has told me he can do no more with medication and he has instructed his staff to locate a movement specialist. Also, my wonderful wife is working with the Veteran's Administration. They will fly Karen and I to and from Houston so we can visit one of their Parkinson's Disease centers of excellence (the VA is setting up six or seven of these centers nationally). They have already bought me a power chair, a regular wheel chair, a power lift to get the chair into and out of the SUV, and hearing aids for both ears. Since I was exposed to Agent Orange when I was an infantry adviser, I may receive 100 percent compensation, too.

May 12, 2011—
Activities/Veteran's Administration

I hope you had a great Easter. Karen and I went to Houston for a visit with PD experts from the Veteran's Administration. We spent three days. The VA paid for air flights to and from Houston; they also paid for the hotel and all medical tests.

I have not been happy with the drugs prescribed by my current neurologist. I have been quite pleased with Dr. Sarwar with the Houston VA. Maybe that was because she agreed with me! Surprise, surprise. She added much to our discussion. She also returned our phone calls, which was great. We agreed to cut back on several drugs.

They did another cognitive thinking test on me and I have slowed a little from the last test, which was three years ago. I must be getting old. But I can remember how old I am: 66.

Several trip highlights:

As we stayed in the VA hospital several nights, we shared a bathroom with a fellow that weighed at least 450 pounds. He was going to have a colonoscopy, and we arrived there the day he was doing his "cleansing process." Glad my nose is not working. Karen wished her nose wasn't working during this ordeal.

However, the true high point was dinner with Frank Jordan, our brother-in-law. A really nice fellow. Super enjoyable. We ate at Papasito's.

The VA made all the travel arrangements and we were assisted by all airport porters.

I am doing physical rehab, which is worthwhile, but my two torn rotator cuffs limit my achievement in arm strength. I asked my physical therapist (PT) here in Bartlesville how did I compare with others who had PD for 12 years. The answer: They all were in a nursing home facility. Currently, I'm being visited twice a week by a PT—once a week by a nurse and once a week by a speech therapist. We will probably up that to several times a week as I try the Lee Silverman LOUD program designed for those with PD to assist with swallowing, strengthening the diaphragm, and improving voice clarity and volume. We hear that my peers have issues with pneumonia, so we are doing all we can to ensure that this won't happen to me.

I stay active with the school board as a community volunteer on the facility committee.

The Oklahoma State University Boone Pickens matching fundraiser will increase the Lowe Family Young Scholars Foundation scholarship endowment fund by $168,000. The sum of $68,000 was received from new donors, and $100,000 more came from T. Boone Pickens post-testament. This will allow us to provide three to four annual scholarships per year to OSU.

An interesting note on the DBS that was performed on me: They were still in the research stage, and I knew that, so you never know what card you will draw next. It seems that they had two options for placing the probes. Apparently, I drew a low card. Now, we are considering removing the two battery boxes the next time when the batteries are ready for replacement. I performed better with my speech when the boxes were turned off at my recent VA appointment. The positioning could also be affecting my cognition. I asked about removing the leads and I was told this was too dangerous. It was not too dangerous to put them in! But I will stay with the research program as long as I can.

Lastly, I think I have developed a black and blue discoloration of my skin over one of the mechanical devices (battery boxes for DBS). Could it be from the recent physical therapy? Is it leaking?

I mentioned earlier, I am feeling better recently. I attribute this to the following: 1) taking the pills always on time, and 2) taking them on an empty stomach. I am adjusting meals along the way.

July 7, 2011—Correspondence
From: Rod

Barry, I so appreciate your sense of dignity, your sense of purpose and your sense of humor. I have tremendous respect for how you have chosen to communicate your situation in stark reality but with a sense of humor. Karen is a huge hero as well, as I think about how she has served you during this time. This e-mail encouraged me mightily.

From: Sheryl

Barry, I can't tell you how much I appreciate you for sharing this journey in your e-mails. We must each face "that lonesome valley" one day. It is less scary when we can share the walk and see the way the Lord has carried His child. I know a lot of your writing is for the purpose of clarifying your own thoughts, and that is also a great example I hope to follow. God bless you and Karen. Many people value your legacy. We are blessed to be your friends.

From: Randy

I can't begin to express all that I feel. Love and respect don't seem enough. Perhaps if I added deep respect and admiration might come close. You are very special!

From: Bobbe

You are in my prayers—as always. I appreciate your updates and thoughts on various subjects. It is amazing that you let us in so completely to your journey. It is brave and unselfish and we appreciate you. You are right. "It's not over till it's over."

July 17, 2011—Family Relationships

This will be a short note. It has been some time since I mentioned that my family is very familiar with PD. My father, my sister, a paternal uncle, and a maternal uncle have or had PD. This concerns my sister, who started with PD five years before me. She has terrible constipation. On the 20th of this month, she is scheduled to have her colon removed.

July 23, 2011—Family Relationships

I just received a phone call from my niece, Michelle, and she said her mother had a heart attack this evening and she didn't make it.

I thank you for your prayers and kind thoughts.

I have had a very busy week. First, I want to thank everyone who prayed for my sister, Sharon. She suffered a long time with her PD. As a friend said: "Siblings have a special relationship because they learn about the world at the same time and they draw strength and compassion for each other … they understand." I will miss her. More later.

July 27, 2011—Correspondence
From: Malinda

I want you to know I am praying for you when I go to bed at night and before I get out of bed in the mornings.

Blessings to you.

July 29, 2011—
Functional Ability/Personal Reflections

Well, today was very interesting. We had our initial meeting with another neurologist. After the session, I went to the men's room. It was not ADA-designed for wheel chairs. In fact, I was trapped for about ten minutes. I asked about ten people who walked by to help me with the doors. No one answered my calls.

As we were driving north, Karen said the doctor asked her several questions: Does your husband know he is in the final stages of PD? Is he getting ready? Does he know he doesn't have much time left? Are his financial records up-to-date? Is his will and trust up to date? Has he checked with hospice? The answer was "yes" to all but the last question.

I accepted this idea about dying about six months ago. I was moving forward rather rapidly through the five stages. In fact, I gave you all a clue. Did you get it? I guess God has decided to bring me home. My work is done. I tried to give Him credit for the good results of the school board and the Lowe Family Young Scholars Program. When I look back, it appears my work at the school board, as founder and fire chief of Columbia Lakes Fire department, and even the US Army combat experience in Vietnam were exposing me to skills I would need to be successful in education and this would not have been possible had not the Lord put Karen and I together. She is a great detail person and she loves kids. We have sent three students to college thus far and 16 are are in the program. We have altered the future for these students.

I must recognize my best friend, Bill Woodard. He was the only person that befriended me during a very difficult time in my career with Phillips. When I had surgery on my back, he went to the hospital and sat with Kris until surgeons said I was okay. Even now, when a degenerative disease like PD slowly sucks the life out of a person, he blocks out an afternoon each week where he repairs items that require attention in the house; we also play dominoes. He is a very smart person, so I felt really good when I tied one match at 200. There is no doubt that Saint Peter will welcome him through the Pearly Gates to heaven when his time comes.

I must mention two other gentlemen: Mike Davis and Charlie Hendricks (Charlie passed away December 24, 2011), who constantly volunteered to help me with anything. The three of us were on the American Legion Honor Guard together. I consider it to be an honor to be associated with such fine men.

There is so much more I want to say. I hope the Lord will give me some time to make a decent book.

They finally operated on my sister July 29. We were told the surgery went well. They sent her home two days later. She had a heart attack and died in the arms of the man she loved and was married to for over 50 years. I called the two nights and weekend before the surgery. As siblings, we were pretty close. She will be missed.

A major decision was whether I should go to Pennsylvania for the funeral. A trip to Tulsa and back really wears me out. Then we found out that she wanted to be cremated and any service would be brief, so I decided to stay home. These decisions are difficult and are easily second guessed.

I mentioned before that my sister had planned to have her colon removed. This is because she had constipation for 20 days many times. This was caused by the drugs she was taking for PD. When it looks like I will go three days without a bowel movement, I start lactulose the second day. I tried six drugs before this one finally worked.

The trouble is, when it works, it usually works ... right now ... so it cannot be taken when I have a busy day. "Excuse me, I must put on a new diaper" doesn't go over well at dinner parties.

To change the subject, an acquaintance recommended I contact a Dr. Ray Marshall in Tulsa. He heals by working on the upper spine. He says the top vertebrae that connect the spine to the brain stem must be in alignment as all nerves must pass through these vertebrae. My connection was 7.5 percent off, blocking 89–90 percent of the signals to and from the brain. I have had two treatments. The jury is still out. More on this next time.

Also, I will share with you how the commode affects constipation. Remember that you heard it here first!

By the way, I have received a 100 percent disability rating from the VA due to Agent Orange exposure which entitles me to free drugs, $2,900 per month and includes things such as home remodeling. You must ask for these benefits and Karen is great at asking.

And lastly, my nurse and I disagree with the neurologist's prediction of my future (regarding hospice).

July 30, 2011—Correspondence
From: Virginia

Oh no, please don't leave me. You are the only person in the world who has known me all my life right from birth. We are just months apart. You found me in 2003 and reconnecting with you has been a true highlight. You are a real relative, not a surrogate I've met along life's journey.

I've been in denial regarding your illness even though I read between the lines in your e-mails. You are such a commanding and strong individual that I guess I assumed you would last forever. However, I am not at all convinced that the end is near.

It is tragic about Sharon, very sudden and unexpected. You were wise not to attempt the long trip. It was very callous of those men to leave you trapped in the men's room. What were they thinking?

I am so happy I came to visit you this time last year. Just to see your surroundings and be with you was wonderful. I so wanted to meet Melissa whom I've become very close with since Kris died. We keep in touch often.

I can't write anymore right now, but will continue later. I'm so sad.

I'm proud of you. I admire you and I love you. I always have.

August 13, 2011—
Medical Condition/Parkinson's Information

I've been getting physical therapy two to three times per week. It stops this week. Now I have a therapist who is telling me how to eat. For example, if I drink liquids, I can only drink 1/3 teaspoon at a time. I cannot eat cereal with milk because I cannot have slurries (for you nonchemical engineers, a slurry is a mixture, not a solution). I am not supposed to eat anything with a straw. This gives early warning if I'm heading for pneumonia.

They have a real piece of technology—they use an X-ray machine that tracks food as it travels from your mouth to your stomach. If you don't swallow correctly, food particles will go to your lungs, causing pneumonia. Why is this important? The number one killer of people with PD is pneumonia.

We hire part-time help for me now. We have a junior at OWU, majoring in nursing, who does a 10:30 p.m. to 8:30 a.m. shift so I can get into and out of bed. Finally, found something that Karen cannot lick. I need 24/7 coverage when Karen goes with her mother to visit Karen's daughter in Kentucky.

Today is one of the best days in some time. I figured it would be a good time to write. Remember not to have rotator cuff breakdown if you have PD. Eldercare loaned a cart to us. That was very nice.

The last update was a little somber. I promised more of an update on research and will do that, but first a comment from Vincent N. Gattullo [president of the American Parkinson Disease Assn.]:

What does it mean to be a Parkinsonian? Well, it means being honest with yourself and your loved ones and facing the truth of your diagnosis and prognosis. It means being brave. Dipping deep within yourself for the inner strength to meet the demands of each day at the highest level you can. It means being humble—accepting the help of your physicians, your family and friends and organizations like APDA, who want to support you and make your life as full as possible. It means being hopeful—knowing that if you must have PD this is the best time to have it—as science understand more about the disease than ever before and is closer to finding a cure.

Azilect

This is from 2006, but is critical knowledge: Azilect has shown in clinical trials that it is highly effective in relieving symptoms with both early and late stages of the disease.

Azilect comes from a class of drugs that can cause dangerous interactions including sudden and severe rises in blood pressure that may lead to stroke and death when patients consume food or drinks that contain a substance found in beer, salami, aged cheeses, soy sauce, and others. It is a tough decision. I believe this is the only drug that works on PD that has been approved since 1973 [which was when carbidopa/levodopa was approved]. I was the only patient in my doctor's entire practice that thought Azilect was worth the risk.

Drug Interaction

Amantadine may interact with Artane. Combined used of these drugs may result in confusion, hallucinations, dry mouth, retention of urine, impotence, blurred vision, dry eyes, abnormal heart beat, flushing of the face and neck, headache and dizziness. I was prescribed to take Artane and amantadine at the same time.

Pesticides

As reported by www.independent.co.uk, research was conducted on 113 people. Out of these, 48 were healthy, 45 had PD, while 20 had Alzheimer's. People with PD (45) had significantly higher levels of pesticides in their body.

I never wore gloves when I was working in the yard, killing fire ants with chemicals that were banned by the FDA. I stored up Dursban because it was so effective. To all who read this, please wear gloves. One dummy is enough.

Personal Update

Finally, I will close with a little personal wisdom. As I mentioned, I finally realized I am going to be in a wheelchair more often than not. When sitting in a chair or lying in bed, it can creep upon me. I take two steps and get the stutter two-steps, but there is nothing to grab onto.

Even though we are changing our home to create a third master bedroom and bath on the first floor that will include my office, I realized I could still fall and that could be it. So, my good friend Mike found a really good scooter for $400 and Karen's dad, Bud, found another chair with a hoist for $500. I bought them both, as Medicare paid $3,850 for a third. I will use one upstairs, one downstairs, and one outside where it will stay and not track in mud for my already-overworked caregiver. I have significantly reduced anxiety with the power chair.

The Stalevo pills work sometimes and sometimes they don't. The doctor said I was in fifth stage and my physical condition should not get much worse. That is the good news. That bad news is when your mental capabilities go south, approximately 40 percent get dementia and 35 percent get Alzheimer's.

August 14, 2011—Living Accommodations

On my front, I was told that hospice joins the team with 60 days left. On June 26 a doctor asked me if I had checked with hospice. The answer was and still is no. It is now August 13, or Day 47. I plan on winning this game Big Time. [Actually, hospice services start at six months, not 60 days. This is clarified in a later entry.]

I have been doing a lot of reading in the years since the doctors agreed with my diagnosis that I had PD. It seemed to me that constipation was always mentioned as a side effect when PD was the main topic. It is thought that Sinemet (the best drug for PD, which was discovered in 1973) was absorbed into the body via the small intestine. This means, of course, it must get into and through the stomach. But, if you are constipated most of the time, this cannot happen. It sounds pretty simple to me. If you have had this condition for several days, it will require much muscle contraction to move that material through the colon. It requires some real grunting and I believe the potential for a heart attack is present. I have tried many drugs (Fibercon and Amitiza to name a few). Lactulose works the best for me.

I read one article that seemed to agree with me, but it bemoaned the fact that almost no research proposals addressed this relationship because it just doesn't sound like serious research. It is difficult to make the topic sound technical. Using words like "feces" and "excrement" doesn't work either, so we are on our own.

I did find an interesting fix that has helped me. We were remodeling our home and were putting in a downstairs full bath. Our home now has four full baths. I realized that I could do my business more efficiently, depending on location. Being a common sense engineer, I measured the height of the commodes and the distance from the floor to the sitting surface. They were very different—14½ inches and 17 inches. If you have short legs and you were using a tall appliance, your toes were just barely touching the floor. Just imagine how the angles of your colon change and the different positions of your buttocks. Well, enough of this jocularity. With my 29 inch legs, I changed to the 14½-inch-tall ivory goddess. Things "work out" much better. If you haven't received two or three chuckles out of this paragraph, you need to loosen up. There's another one!

September 2, 2011—
Emergency Room Visit/Chiropractic Care

As far as falling is concerned, my last fall was on June 20. That is 108 days without a fall. The statistics look good, but as someone always says, statistics lie.

I was taken to the emergency room on Saturday evening at Karen's insistence. I thought I was in an extended down cycle but I sweated all over the bed. Then I became cold and my teeth were chattering. To make a long story short, I had a urinary tract infection. According to the literature it is extremely dangerous for PD folks due to our low immune system. They gave me antibiotics for a week to combat the urinary tract infection and said I should be okay in a week. If not, I would need a second week of pills.

It seems that these antibiotics kill all bacteria, both good and bad, so they must select the antibiotic very carefully for a PD patient. It was determined that I had Thrush. More on this later.

The story continues. I asked what caused the urinary tract infection. There is no standard answer, as it is very unusual, but I put my little used engineering brain to work. Sic 'em, Rover.

I believe the external catheter was the culprit. When you put it on, you can very easily twist the soft rubber tube on the catheter. So when you try to urinate, this restriction forces the urine back to where it came from—the bladder.

According to a caretaker blog, http://www.myparkinsons. org, you can prevent a urinary tract infection by taking a specific natural cranberry extract each and every day. "A UTI in any senior citizen is a nightmare. The toxins from the bacteria do not clear the system very quickly and end up congregating in the brain, the very worst place. The person becomes disoriented, confused, and delusional. It is very scary. In a senior PD person, it is worse."

Upon my doctor's follow-up visit, they found bilirubin in my urine. It is an alert that your liver might be malfunctioning, so back in for another test. The test said I was okay, but I needed to eat more protein. But, I am not supposed to eat much protein for the Sinemet to be effective! What is the old saying? "You get it coming or going."

The good news is that cranberry juice can completely prevent a urinary tract infection. Once you have the UTI, drinking cranberry juice will do nothing, so you have to drink it every day to be preventative. Taking cranberry pills is cost effective and it gives good results. It is recommended to use Spring Valley, triple strength cranberry fruit 2,000 mg, twice a day. They can be purchased at Wal-Mart.

I have mentioned previously a drug called Neupro. It is efficiently and effectively delivered through the skin; however, it is not available in the United States due to an FDA ruling. [Newpro is available in the U.S. as of June, 2012.] The generic drug name is rotigotine. Well, we found a way to get it through a manufacturer in the UK who transports it through Canada as a home health care item. The advantage of the patch is that it gives a more constant drug dosage. There are fewer lows, and the lows are not as deep. Each patch has 2 mg of rotigotine. I believe this drug allows us to extend the wearing off of Sinemet's effectiveness, and that is very important. The effectiveness of Sinemet is normally around seven years, and if you use large quantities of Sinemet, it will not last that long. World class doctors disagree greatly on this issue. I was taking 3,000 mg per day; the prescription was approved by three neurologists. But after DBS, the new doctor cut me immediately to 1,000 mg maximum. Most literature suggests 600 mg maximum. Please remember that these examples are my perception of my case. I am not a doctor.

Also, we decided to check into a chiropractor [Dr. Ray mentioned earlier] who seems to be able to cure folks of various illnesses or their side effects. His hands never touch (or may lightly touch) your body and the treatments take about 20 seconds and cost $40 per visit. My last neurologist charged $600 for the visit. Dr. Ray took three X-rays and determined that my upper spine was 7.5 degrees out of alignment with my brain stem. He had me lie on my side and after he finished in less than one minute, he told me I could get up. And I did. I was amazed. I was very rigid at the time. Switching out my Neupro on a daily basis and having a weekly visit to my chiropractor allows me to feel pretty good for the past two weeks. And then I started heading south.

Next time I will provide a review of my daily pill requirements.

September 22, 2011— Medications/Living with Parkinson's

In the last status report, I said I would list the drugs that have been prescribed for me. I will not list the dosage or the number of doses per day because I am certain they will change, dependent upon the patient's history and the stage of PD they are in. Doctors make these decisions, but the doctors, especially neurologists, have very different thoughts on how they will treat a person. For example, my sister took 800 mg per day of Sinemet and I took 3,000+ mg of the same drug plus Azilect.

Current list: carbidopa/levodopa (Sinemet), Clonazepam, cyanocobalamin shots (B12), enalapril (Lotrel), entacapone, etodolac (replaced Celebrex), lactulose, Azilect (rasagiline), Claritin (loratadine), Mucinex (guaifenesin), Neupro (rotigotine), Provigil (modafinil), vitamin D3, amlodipine besylate, quetiapine furmate (Seroquel), selenium, saw palmetto, cranberry pills.

At least four of these pills are in excess of $500 per month in the retail market. The cost is $8 per month through the VA.

A few corrections from the last report. Hospice is normally called in when a patient is estimated to have six months to live, not 60 days as I mentioned earlier. On June 26, 2011, it was suggested that I check with hospice. The answer was and still is no. Six months from June 26 will be Christmas.

Also, I stopped my fall record. I fell on Tuesday, September 19, 2011. I was in the front yard and tripped on a magnolia tree ground root. I tried to knock down my neighbor's rock wall—face first. I went by ambulance to the ER, where I am on a first name basis with employees. I do get to add this to my injury list from falls in the past 18 months: six stitches in my upper lip.

Previous injuries received from falls include the following:

- Two torn rotator cuffs

- Two dislocated thumbs

- A dislocated shoulder

- Four broken ribs

- A brain hemorrhage requiring emergency surgery

- A forehead injury requiring 20 stitches and five clamps (split my head open)

- An arm injury requiring five stitches

Several readers have suggested I use the status reports as the basis for a book. I have contacted a few publishers and the typing is underway. Suggestions are very welcome.

October 9, 2011—Medical Care/Planning

I have really abused my falling records. I had one fall in the house that resulted in approximately 30 stitches and a fall in the yard that resulted in a busted lip and six more stitches. On the good side, I am letting my hair become a mustache—and Karen likes it!

I learned more about being a doctor. They treated me with antibiotics, but that must be done very carefully because it kills both bad and good bacteria. Karen saw a strange growth on my tongue after taking antibiotics. In effect, my body was being attacked by two bugs. Several doctors and nurses did not see this, but Karen did. If you have PD, your immune system is already weakened and you must be extra careful. Guess I better keep her. She contacted our home care nurse (sent her a picture via her mobile phone), who quickly diagnosed it as thrush and called the doctor. He prescribed meds immediately. Technology is really wonderful sometimes!

It was time for my periodic prostate check. I cut back on selenium and flaxseed oil when I lowered my PSA count by a full point to 3.5. It rose again to 4.5. The doctor said the prostate was enlarged but had no soft spots, and we will go to the six-month PSA tests. The PSA test gives 50 percent false positives, and with my recent fevers, I am glad the doctor did not recommend a biopsy.

I believe I had mentioned that my B12 level was too low and it is responsible for maintaining the spine's immune system. I now take one B12 shot per week, and I have reintroduced selenium and flaxseed oil into my pill regimen. They make it so you really want the B12 shot, as the needle is 1½ inches long; it does get your attention.

Our new neurologist gave us a prescription for Neupro, a patch-type drug which decreases the cyclic lows of PD. It is a 24-hour transdermal patch, but you cannot buy it in the States due to the FDA. I complained to our new neurologist about this, and he said I needed to write to the government. I told him I wrote to Senator Coburn; he said he had also.

He gave me a prescription and Karen purchased the drug from a Canadian firm. It was manufactured in England.

By the way, a friend gave me an article that was entitled "New and Exciting Ways to Treat PD," from a *RealCures* pamphlet by Dr. Frank Shallenberger. I read the five-page article and was concerned that only one patient was used in a published study. Dr. Marty Hinz is the lead researcher. If the case study was published, and if the treatment cured PD, they would have to build a Wal-Mart-type parking lot next to the doctor's office. In addition, I asked Dr. Piper, the President of the Oklahoma Wesleyan University campus in Bartlesville, Oklahoma, if he had a chemistry professor who would review this for me. He did, and the professor agreed with me on the minimal review and two additional points.

The professor also recommended I read a book recently published by one of the world's leading immunologists, Dr. T.

Colin Campbell. It is entitled *The China Study*. It is focused on dietary control to offset illness, and it validates a vegan diet.

I do not currently plan to try Dr. Hinz's plan, but as my options disappear, who knows. I will let you all know before I give it a go.

I am seeing another doctor who performs neck adjustments for 10–15 seconds. The first time I had been lying on a six-inch-tall table. After he was done, he said, "I'm finished." I easily stood up. What a surprise. The follow-up treatments only cost $40—much more cost efficient than the drugs that cost $140 per month. I plan to continue this treatment for now.

Many readers have encouraged me to write a book that will contain answers to a lot of their questions. It will include my humor and the events that provide flashbacks that show life must go on. You just have to make it so. I tell friends that I used to work 12 hours per day, but now the PD restricts me to three to four hours per day.

My typing finger has a blister on it, so it is time to stop. Treat each day as it might be your last; treat people the same way.

When fighting in Vietnam, I thought I might not survive, but little did I know that my biggest adversary came home with me. Now I fight my biggest battle, here on home soil, against "Mr. P."

Conclusion

This book has two potential endings. The first tracks the epigraph quote from Harper Lee at the front of this book, but let's end this story on a positive and motivating note. We will be optimistic and decide that a miracle drug is discovered and it actually cures the disease. Also, we have been following these Best Practices:

1. If you have Parkinson's, always take your pills on schedule. This is very important and more difficult than a novice might think. If I were two hours late, almost a full cycle, it would take a full day to get to normal again. It is critical that you meet this requirement. The impact is very severe, and the more advanced your Parkinson's is, the more important. You can purchase watches that vibrate on six settings. This helps for awhile.

2. Adjust your meals so your stomach has no protein to

be absorbed in conflict with levodopa absorption. I finally decided it was better to miss a meal than to eat a Quarter Pounder before taking the meds.

3. Exercise is a double-edged sword. As your disease becomes more advanced, exercise will use up the levodopa sooner and your cycles will become shorter.

4. Remember that Sinemet is the best med to slow down Parkinson's advancement, and nothing better has been made available since 1973. Sinemet is not a cure.

5. You must accept the fact that you will wake up every morning and the disease will still be there and it will be a little worse. Your good hours become less as you move thru the five stages. As the good hours become reduced they become more precious and you must use them to make your life richer and more rewarding.

6. Individuals will pass through the five stages at different speeds. As you go up in stages, I would expect your meds to increase. Be alert—the five stages are only approximate physical changes. They do not try to estimate mental changes.

7. Remember there is no single accepted methodology to treat Parkinson's, so when you change doctors do not be surprised if your stash of meds for emergencies becomes worthless.

8. Many drugs try to extend the effectiveness of Sinemet. Some of the drugs are Requip, Azilect, Mirapex, Comtan, Stalevo, and Neupro. I will not try to explain the different mechanisms that the medical

community believes actually happen, because it is too technical for my simple mind to understand. I can tell you, however, that there is now a new theory that meds may work at one stage but not another. For example, I was trying Neupro before the FDA stopped that drug from being purchased in the United States. That didn't bother me, as I was receiving little benefit. Yet as I tracked the meds, it became apparent to me that I had a thin threshold between when I was feeling really good and really bad. Neupro was noted for removing most of the "low" lows and the "high" highs. Consequently, Neupro fit the bill to my threshold issues, but we could not buy it in the United States. We were able to obtain a prescription for Neupro that is available internationally but not in the United States. It works well for me.

9. There is a major disagreement on how much Sinemet a patient should take per day. The range is from 1,050 mg per day to 800 mg per day. I was up to 3,050 mg per day prior to DBS and 850 mg per day after DBS. I am currently at 1,200 mg per day with help from Neupro and Azilect, and I'm currently investigating Comtan.

10. Remember that DBS works best on tremors, not stiffness. I have never had tremors.

11. If you have DBS surgery, you will be awake during the 4½-hour procedure. You will hear it all. I will always remember the words, "Hurry! Irrigate that quickly." The Velcro cocoon is a very memorable experience as well.

12. Remember that *you are still alive.* Go places, do things!

13. Remember your caregiver. They will carry your message forward—whether good or bad.

14. Read your prescription.

15. Research on the Internet.

16. Read the vendor information.

Take care,
Barry

Author Biography

Barry W. Lowe was born in 1945 to Wilbur and Grace Lowe. He had one sister and one brother. His sister died of a Parkinson's-related heart attack on July 24, 2011. His father had Parkinson's, as did a paternal uncle and a maternal uncle. Barry was an Honor Graduate of the US Army's Basic Officer's Course. He volunteered for service as an infantry adviser in Vietnam in 1969. He was awarded the Bronze Star and the Combat Infantry Badge and the Expert badge for the M-16 rifle. He is on 100 percent disability as a result of his service to his country. He was familiar with the use of Agent Orange. He earned a chemical engineering bachelor's degree at Lafayette University and an MBA at Oklahoma State University. While at Oklahoma State, he was inducted into two academic fraternities, Phi Kappa Phi and Beta Sigma Phi.

He worked for Proctor and Gamble in operations. In 1974, he joined Phillips Petroleum Company and had management positions in construction, operations, research and development, process design, and project management. When he retired in 2000, his division had responsibility for cost estimates, planning and scheduling and project management worldwide.

Awards and Honors

The American Institute of Chemical Engineers National Recognition Award of 1987.

The American Institute of Chemical Engineers National Membership Award of 1987.

The state of Oklahoma Society School Board Association Buddy Spencer Leadership Award in 2006

The Oklahoma All-state all star Board of Education in 2006.

The AARP Oklahoma Top 50 award in 2010.

The Oklahoma Making a Difference Award in Education in 2003.

The Bartlesville Civitan Citizen of the year award in 2007.

The Ray Steiner Champions Award from the Big Brothers— Big Sisters Award in 2009.

The Bartlesville League of Women Voters Citizen of the year award in 2011.

The Most Progressive Citizen of Bartlesville in 2008.

The Rotary Paul Harris Fellow Award in 2002.